Updates in Surgery

Nicolò de Manzini
Editor

Rectal Cancer

Strategy and Surgical Techniques

Forewords by
Gianluigi Melotti
Christian Meyer

Springer

Editor
Nicolò de Manzini
Department of Medicine, Surgery and Health Sciences
General Surgery Unit
Cattinara University Hospital
Trieste, Italy

The publication and the distribution of this volume have been supported by the Italian Society of Surgery

ISSN 2280-9848
ISBN 978-88-470-5837-8 ISBN 978-88-470-2670-4 (eBook)

DOI 10.1007/978-88-470-2670-4

Springer Milan Dordrecht Heidelberg London New York

Softcover re-print of the Hardcover 1st edition 2013

9 8 7 6 5 4 3 2 1 2013 2014 2015 2016

Cover design: Ikona S.r.l., Milan, Italy
Typesetting: Graphostudio, Milan, Italy

Springer-Verlag Italia S.r.l. – Via Decembrio 28 – I-20137 Milan
Springer is a part of Springer Science+Business Media (www.springer.com)

Foreword

Rectal cancer has become an increasingly common disease in Western countries, largely because of lifestyle and nutritional factors. While mortality has fallen since the 1980s owing to earlier diagnosis and improved therapy, the disease not only continues to pose a threat to survival but also impacts markedly on quality of life. Greater understanding of all aspects of the disease and a full appreciation of the still evolving role of surgery will be essential in achieving further progress.

This volume, by Nicolò de Manzini and his collaborators, will without doubt make a superb contribution in communicating state of the art knowledge on this serious disease and in particular in explaining clearly current surgical strategy and techniques. In so doing, it will not only fulfil the aim of the Società Italiana di Chirurgia (Italian Society of Surgery) to disseminate such knowledge but also showcase the excellent standards of Italian surgery.

The authors take great pains to describe the various available surgical techniques in the meticulous detail required by surgeons in training, and fully address important related aspects such as salvage situations, accidents, complications, and their treatment. This is not, however, simply a book on surgery. Diagnosis and staging, pathology, molecular evaluation, and follow-up are all covered clearly and convincingly, with helpful explanation of the links to the therapeutic options.

Professor de Manzini is to be congratulated on the high quality that he has successfully striven to achieve throughout the work. In ensuring that all aspects of rectal cancer and its surgical treatment are covered in an interrelated and fully up to date manner, he has produced a most instructive book that will prove an invaluable asset for the surgical community.

Rome, September 2012

Gianluigi Melotti
President, Italian Society of Surgery

Foreword

In economically developed countries, improvements in the standard of living have increased life expectancy, mainly due to high-quality healthcare. Nonetheless, the other side of the coin is that progress achieved in public health has been challenged by new threats such as cancer, commonly including malignancies involving the lower bowel. Rectal cancer, in particular, accounts for more than one third of colorectal cancers. These patients suffer severe side effects of the disease and have a poor prognosis. Moreover, they are frequently confronted with a very painful infirmity, often necessitating the creation of a digestive stoma with all its physical and psychological implications.

At the same time, due to tireless research efforts and worldwide sharing of best practices over the last 20 years, there have been several therapeutic breakthroughs, bringing about some bright patches in a despairingly dark sky. Thus, today we can state that in three out of four patients with rectal cancers who undergo surgery the integrity of the sphincter system can be preserved, thus reversing the situation most common 30 years ago.

This extraordinary result reflects, on the one hand, improvements in radiological investigations prior to therapy, allowing better definition of cancer staging and the selection of patients who might require neo adjuvant radiochemotherapy, and, on the other hand, the tremendous evolution in surgical techniques, including ultra-low colo-anal anastomoses. This procedure is usually considered as major surgery because of the difficult postoperative period. Therefore, in the last 10 years, surgeons have made enormous endeavors to reduce the postoperative impact by using minimally invasive techniques as often as possible, mostly laparoscopy but also trans-anal endoscopic exeresis. This approach, which represents significant advances in surgical know-how, demands great skill and considerable experience.

As a step forward in one area depends on and leads to improvements in many others, contributions by other disciplines have become an essential aspect, both anatomically and pathologically, with respect to refinements in cancer-staging procedures and thus a better forecast of outcomes. These developments have been accompanied by discoveries in the oncologic genetics and molecular biology of tumor resistance to chemotherapeutic agents.

These topics and many others are comprehensively discussed in this outstanding volume. The information is presented in clearly written chapters supported by high-quality figures and tables as well as up-to-date references derived from the world literature.

This monograph, edited and co-authored by Professor Nicolò de Manzini, Head of the Surgical Department of the University of Trieste, has been written in close cooperation with experts in related disciplines and testifies to the energy of the Trieste school of surgery. Thus, the volume is not merely a theoretical analysis sustained by the literature, it also draws on the strong clinical knowledge and experience of the authors.

This impressive volume deserves to be widely diffused and certainly merits a place of honor on the bookshelf of every surgeon and oncologist, who in treating these patients will benefit from its state-of-the-art approach.

Strasbourg, September 2012

Christian Meyer
Emeritus Professor
Strasbourg University Hospital

Preface

Rectal cancer is a frequent neoplasm in Western countries, mainly due to dietary and environmental factors. Its serious impact derives not only from the poor prognosis, but also from the important sequelae potentially provoked by its treatment. Over the last three decades, the management of rectal cancer has changed, reflecting better knowledge of the anatomy of the pelvis, a refinement of surgical technique to yield improved oncological and functional results, and advances in neoadjuvant and adjuvant therapy. In fact, current therapeutic strategy takes into account the tumor's response to neoadjuvant therapy and the status of pelvic functions. The concepts of oncological radicality and sphincter-saving have led to a strong emphasis on sphincter preservation through intersphincteric resections, such that the pathological response may allow a shift towards rectal-saving procedures. Translating these considerations into practice will most likely call for a multidisciplinary approach in order to define the optimal strategy, which in frequent cases will be tailored to the patient.

This volume provides an up-to-date discussion of several aspects of rectal cancer, from a theoretical as well as a practical point of view.

The first part begins with an analysis of the epidemiology of rectal cancer and then moves on to address imaging of this disease, its pathology, and its molecular markers, concluding with the roles of the various imaging modalities and the results obtained with radiochemotherapy.

The second part focuses on therapeutically aimed surgical procedures, including perioperative management and the different steps of the various operations, especially laparoscopic access. Reconstruction, nerve-sparing options, the role of stomas, and intra-and postoperative problems are reviewed in separate chapters.

There is also a chapter devoted to multimodal strategies, and another in which current problems in the follow-up of patients with rectal cancer and the strategies for the treatment of local relapse are investigated.

We hope that this broad panorama is able to convey the knowledge required for the proper diagnosis and management of rectal cancer.

Finally, we thank Laura Zicari for the anatomical drawings, Giancarlo Pengo for the photographic processing and Malcolm Clark for the English translation.

Trieste, September 2012 Nicolò de Manzini

Contents

Contributors

Alessandro Carrer Molecular Medicine Laboratory, International Centre for Genetic Engineering and Biotechnology (ICGEB), Trieste, Italy

Biagio Casagranda Department of Medicine, Surgery and Health Sciences, General Surgery Unit, Cattinara University Hospital, Trieste, Italy

Roberta Cavallin Department of Medicine, Surgery and Health Sciences, General Surgery Unit, Cattinara University Hospital, Trieste, Italy

Davide Cosola Department of Medicine, Surgery and Health Sciences, General Surgery Unit, Cattinara University Hospital, Trieste, Italy

Maria Assunta Cova Department of Medicine, Surgery and Health Sciences, Radiology Unit, Cattinara University Hospital, Trieste, Italy

Nicolò de Manzini Department of Medicine, Surgery and Health Sciences, General Surgery Unit, Cattinara University Hospital, Trieste, Italy

Luca De Paoli Department of Medicine, Surgery and Health Sciences, Radiology Unit, Cattinara University Hospital, Trieste, Italy

Alessandro De Pellegrin Department of Medicine, Surgery and Health Sciences, Pathology Unit, Cattinara University Hospital, Trieste, Italy

Massimo Giacca Department of Medicine, Surgery and Health Sciences, General Surgery Unit, Cattinara University Hospital, Trieste, Italy

Mauro Giacca Molecular Medicine Laboratory, International Centre for Genetic Engineering and Biotechnology (ICGEB), Trieste, Italy and Department of Medical, Surgical and Health Sciences, University of Trieste, Italy

Greta Giacomel Department of Medicine, Surgery and Health Sciences, General Surgery Unit, Cattinara University Hospital, Trieste, Italy

Michela Giuricin Department of Medicine, Surgery and Health Sciences, General Surgery Unit, Cattinara University Hospital, Trieste, Italy

Paola Graziotin Department of Medicine, Surgery and Health Sciences, General Surgery Unit, Cattinara University Hospital, Trieste, Italy

Alessandra Guglielmi Department of Oncology, "Ospedali Riuniti" University Hospital, Trieste, Italy

Marco Kosuta Department of Medicine, Surgery and Health Sciences, General Surgery Unit, Cattinara University Hospital, Trieste, Italy

Piera Leon Department of Medicine, Surgery and Health Sciences, General Surgery Unit, Cattinara University Hospital, Trieste, Italy

Alessandra Lucchetta Department of Medicine, Surgery and Health Sciences, General Surgery Unit, Cattinara University Hospital, Trieste, Italy

Simonetta Masaro Department of Medicine, Surgery and Health Sciences, General Surgery Unit, Cattinara University Hospital, Trieste, Italy

Elisa Moretti Department of Medicine, Surgery and Health Sciences, General Surgery Unit, Cattinara University Hospital, Trieste, Italy

Silvia Palmisano Department of Medicine, Surgery and Health Sciences, General Surgery Unit, Cattinara University Hospital, Trieste, Italy

Emilio Quaia Department of Medicine, Surgery and Health Sciences, Radiology Unit, Cattinara University Hospital, Trieste, Italy

Andrea Romano Department of Medicine, Surgery and Health Sciences, Pathology Unit, Cattinara University Hospital, Trieste, Italy

Paola Tarchi Department of Medicine, Surgery and Health Sciences, General Surgery Unit, Cattinara University Hospital, Trieste, Italy

Mattia Trevisan Department of Medicine, Surgery and Health Sciences, General Surgery Unit, Cattinara University Hospital, Trieste, Italy

Fabrizio Zanconati Department of Medicine, Surgery and Health Sciences, Pathology Unit, Cattinara University Hospital, Trieste, Italy

Epidemiology

1

Michela Giuricin, Alessandra Lucchetta, Greta Giacomel
and Nicolò de Manzini

1.1 Introduction

This chapter analyzes the epidemiology of rectal cancer, first of all on a global scale, then concentrating on the situation in the USA, with reference to the great number of publications available, and finally looking at the situation in Italy, which the authors are most familiar with.

1.2 World

Colorectal cancer is one of the most frequent neoplastic diseases on a worldwide scale. Seventy-two per cent of these carcinomas arise in the colon and only 28% are rectal; however, from an epidemiological viewpoint the two neoplasms are usually considered together [1, 2]. Of all the neoplasms, colorectal cancer is the third most frequent in men (10%) and in women (9.4%); it is the fourth most common cause of death in males (7.6%) and the third most common in women (8.6%).

Incidence rises with an increase in age in both sexes: in males the mean age of diagnosis is slightly lower than that of women (60-65 years vs. 65-70 years).

It follows the same trend in terms of associated mortality, with an earlier peak in men (65-70 years) compared to women (70-75 years); however, mortality has dropped since the beginning of the 1980s, probably due to earlier diagnosis of the disease as well as to improvements in therapy [1, 3].

M. Giuricin (✉)
Department of Medicine, Surgery and Health Sciences, General Surgery Unit,
Cattinara University Hospital,
Trieste, Italy
e-mail: michelagiuricin@libero.it

N. de Manzini (ed.), *Rectal Cancer,*
Updates in Surgery
DOI: 10.1007/978-88-470-2670-4_1, © Springer-Verlag Italia 2013

Colorectal cancer is more common in developed than in developing countries: 13.1% vs. 7.1%; in the latter area, this carcinoma is only the seventh most common of all neoplasms. Moreover, the death rate from colorectal cancer rises from 11.7% in industrialized countries to 6.3% in developing countries [1].

An analysis of the data on the recto-anal region reported in the 2002 database of the IARC (International Agency for Research on Cancer) shows that as regards women New Zealand occupies first place in the classification, followed by Australia, Israel, Germany, Japan, and Singapore, while with regard to men the same database shows the Czech Republic at the top, followed by Japan, Slovakia, Germany, Australia, France and Slovenia.

For both sexes, Italy is in the bottom half of the classification, and is one of the last of the industrialized countries [4].

1.2.1 USA

In the USA, colorectal cancer is the third most common cancer in both sexes, with a reduction in the last 20 years: from 66.3 cases per 100,000 subjects in 1985 to 45.3 in 2007. The decline accelerated from 1998 to 2007 (2.9% a year for men and 2.2% a year for women), probably thanks to improvements in diagnosis, which allowed an increasing number of polyps to be eradicated earlier than before. A total of 39,870 new cases of rectal cancer was forecast for 2011 [3, 5].

In the period 2004-2008 the average age of diagnosis was 70 years; the rate of incidence was 55 per 100,000 males and 41 per 100,000 women, with a greater incidence in Afro-Americans of both sexes compared to the other races. In the same period, the mortality was 20.7 per 100,000 men and 14.5 per 100,000 women, here too with a preponderance for Afro-Americans [5].

Cancer-related survival at 5 years (2001-2007) was on average 64.3%: 65.5% for males (55% Afro-Americans) and 64.5% for females (56.9% Afro-Americans) [5].

According to the SEER database, in the USA 1 in 20 people are at risk of developing colorectal cancer during their lifetime [6].

In contrast with the global reduction of incidence and mortality, an increase in the incidence of rectal cancer has been found in subjects aged less than 40. The Meyer et al. study published in 2010 shows how 1,922 patients diagnosed with rectal carcinoma between 1973 and 2005 were less than 40 years old; of these 52% were male, 52% were between 35 and 39 years old and 75% were Caucasians. In this period the incidence was 0.42 per 100,000 people, and in time it increased significantly (APC, Annual Percentage Change, 2.6% $p<.0001$), while to the incidence of cancer of the colon remained unchanged (APC -0.2% $p=0.50$). An increase was also found for cancer of the rectosigmoid junction: an incidence of 0.13 per 100,000 subjects, APC 2.2.% $p<.0001$. Sex and age do not affect these data. Subjects younger than 40 in this study also showed higher lymphatic and vascular invasion and a pattern of infiltrative growth, with a consequent more advanced stage and a lower global survival rate than that of older patients. This is probably connected to a slight delay in diagnosis, considering that none of these symptoms alone will necessarily trigger the patient's physician to include malignancy in the differential diagnosis. On the other hand, a study by Schellerer et al. in 2011 revealed how the prognosis in these subjects is comparable to that in over 40 year olds, since multimodal therapy is applicable with an acceptable risk. Furthermore, as under-40s tend to be in better health conditions, they have a lower anesthesiological risk, suffer fewer postoperative complications and tolerate the toxicity of chemotherapy better [7, 8].

1.2.2 Italy

In Italy rectal cancer is the seventh most common neoplasia in both men (3.7% of all cancers) and women (3.3% of the total). These data come from population-based tumor registers (AIRT 1998-2002), which currently cover around a quarter of the Italian population.

Along with true rectal cancer, lesions of the rectosigmoid junction, the anus and the anal canal are included with rectal tumors.

This neoplasia represents 3.1% of all cancer deaths among men and 3.3% among women.

Estimates show a total of 20,457 colorectal tumors among the male population and 17,276 diagnosed annually among women, with a mortality for colorectal cancer in the year 2002 of 2,504 male subjects and 2,052 females.

In the population considered in the Italian registers, an average of 28.6 cases per 100,000 males and 20 per 100,000 females are diagnosed annually, thus showing a significant prevalence among males.

The cumulative lifetime risk of developing rectal cancer (between 0 and 74 years old) is 17.2‰ among men and 9.3‰ among women, while the cumulative mortality risk is 5.3‰ for men and 2.7‰ for women.

Over time colorectal cancer has shown a slight increase in incidence among men, whereas it has remained more or less stable among the female population; mortality has decreased in both sexes.

Adenocarcinomas (67-74%) or malignant tumors NOS (10-11%) are more frequent, while histological diagnosis rarely reveals adenocarcinomas in villous adenomas (4-5%), in adenomatous polyps (2-3%) or mucinous forms (3-5%).

As regards relative survival, the 5-year rate is 54% for men and 56% for women, decreasing with age for men, while in women it is stable or sometimes better up to 64 years of age, subsequently decreasing in percentages comparable with the data for males after 65 years of age.

There is a slight geographical variation in the rectal tumor rate in Italy, with a higher incidence in the northern regions; however, survival is greater in the centre-north regions (53-55%) compared to those of the south (45%). Five-year survival improved from 1985-87 to 2000-2002, from about 43% to 58% [9].

1.2.3 Conclusions

- Colorectal cancer is the third most common neoplasia globally, but is more frequent in industrialized countries or those with growing economies.
- Mortality decreased over the last 20 years, probably thanks to the early eradication of polyps as well as to therapeutic progress.
- In the USA an increase has been found in rectal carcinomas and in subjects under the age of 40.
- In Italy the incidence is increasing slightly in males, whereas mortality is decreasing in both sexes. There is a certain geographical variability, with a greater incidence in the north compared to the centre-south, but mortality is greater in southern regions.

1.3 Risk Factors

Factors increasing the risk of developing colorectal cancer can be modifiable or nonmodifiable.

The latter include hereditary and genetic factors, including familial adenomatous polyposis of the colon, the Lynch syndrome, chronic intestinal inflammatory illnesses, and a previous history of colorectal neoplasia or a family history of it.

Patients with these conditions have almost twice the chance of developing colorectal cancer than the rest of the population, and the earlier the family member developed the tumor, or if several family members have been diagnosed with colorectal neoplasia, the greater the risk [10, 11]. These people are therefore advised to start an endoscopic screening programme at least 10 years earlier than those not at risk.

Non-modifiable factors must also include the "age parameter", as the incidence of rectal cancer increases with age. According to the annual report regarding colorectal cancer trends in the United States from 1975 to 2006 by Edwards et al., more than 90% of cases of colorectal neoplasia are diagnosed in subjects aged over 50, but often when the diagnosis is made in subjects aged less than 50, the neoplasia is at an advanced stage. The incidence of neoplasia at an age of under fifty is higher in black people than in Hispanics, though an increase has been observed amongst American Indians and natives of Alaska [10].

The so-called modifiable risk factors are those involving a habit that can be changed.

Diet seems to have an impact on the probability of developing colorectal cancer. Eating large quantities of red meat and processed meat seems to increase the occurrence of neoplasia. In fact, these foods are full of fats, proteins and heme iron, factors which can promote cancerogenesis; furthermore, processed meat can produce heterocyclic amines and nitrous compounds which are mutagenic agents and carcinogenic substances in animal models [12].

The regular consumption of large amounts of alcohol is reported to be one of the risk factors for the development of neoplasia, rectal cancer in particular, and the risk seems to be directly correlated to the amount consumed [13].

Obesity also seems to be one of the risk factors for rectal neoplasia. A meta-analysis by Larsson and Wolk indicates a correlation between BMI and the incidence of colorectal cancer, which varies according to sex and age: the risk of colon cancer increases with increasing BMI, particularly with android obesity, and especially in males, while the risk of rectal cancer increases with increasing BMI in men, but not in women [14].

A meta-analysis by Harris et al. of 29 studies reviewed also agrees with the above observations regarding the negative relation between BMI and an increased risk of colon cancer in both sexes, and of rectal neoplasia in men alone [15].

The exact mechanism of the correlation between obesity and colorectal cancer is not entirely clear, but hormonal alterations, particularly insulin and insulin-like growth factor (IGF) seem to play a significant role; the hyperinsulinemia present in obese patients determines an increase in free IGF with a consequent modification of the cellular environment in terms of mitogenesis and antiapoptosis, promoting the formation of tumor cells [14, 15].

The last habit linked to an increased risk of developing colorectal carcinoma is smoking. A meta-analysis by Botteri et al. of 106 observational studies highlighted a significant association of smoking with colorectal cancer, both in terms of incidence and in terms of the associated mortality [16]. Paskett et al. compared their own observational study to three clinical trials regarding female smokers, pointing out an increase in the risk of colorectal cancer and particularly rectal cancer; the same study reports that cutting down on smoking may reduce the risk of this disease [17].

Along with the risk factors, those defined as protective factors should also be recalled.

As described in the MISCAN-Colon model, which is also cited in the study by Cuzick et al., the regular use of aspirin seems to be a protective factor in the prevention of some tumors, including colorectal cancer [18]. Different eating habits have been referred to as protective factors, including the consumption of folates, which according to Jaszewski et al. also protect against the recurrence of colorectal adenomas [19, 20]. Alongside folates, the regular intake of other micronutrients in the diet, including calcium and vitamins, are among the factors protecting against the development of colorectal neoplasia, without a precise distinction between colon and rectal neoplasia [10].

Finally, there is an inverse correlation between moderate but regular physical activity and cancer of the colon in both men and women, as evidenced in the review by Harriss et al., but this association was not observed for cancer of the rectum [21].

1.3.1 Conclusions

- There is not always a distinction in literature between the risk factors of colon and of rectal cancer: they are often grouped together.
- Risk factors can be modifiable or non-modifiable. The latter include age and hereditary factors, for which the only form of protection may be to perform genetic studies, or at least early endoscopic examinations.
- On the other hand, risk factors like eating, negative lifestyle habits and physical exercise can be controlled and modified, and are those over which we have some power to prevent the disease. However, no studies have shown a direct correlation between a modifiable factor and colorectal cancer incidence.

References

1. World Health Organization. International Agency for Research on Cancer (IARC) (2011). Available at http://www-dep.iarc.fr/ Accessed December 3, 2011
2. American Cancer Society (2008) Colorectal Cancer Facts & Figures 2008-2010. American Cancer Society, Atlanta
3. American Cancer Society (2011) Cancer Facts & Figures 2011. American Cancer Society, Atlanta
4. Center MM, Jemal A, Smith RA, Ward E (2009) Worldwide variations in Colorectal Cancer. CA Cancer J Clin 59:366-378
5. National Cancer Institute (2011) Rectal Cancer Treatment (PDQ®). http://www.cancer.gov/
6. Surveillance Epidemiology and End Result (SEER) (2011) Stat Fact Sheets: Colon and Rectum. http://seer.cancer.gov/statfacts/html/colorect.html
7 Meyer JE, Narang T, Schnoll-Sussman FH et al (2010) Increasing incidence of rectal cancer in patients aged younger than 40 years. Cancer 116:4354-4359
8 Schellerer VS, Merkel S, Schumann SC et al (2012) Despite aggressive histopathology survival is not impaired in young patients with colorectal cancer. Int J Colorectal Dis 27:71-79
9. Associazione Italiana Registri Tumori (AIRTUM) (2006) Tumore del retto (ICD-10 = C19-21). www.registri-tumori.it
10. Edwards BK, Ward E, Kohler BA et al (2010) Annual report to the nation on the status of cancer, 1975-2006, featuring colorectal cancer trends and impact of interventions (risk factors, screening, and treatment) to reduce future rates. Cancer 116:544-573
11. Lynch HT, de la Chapelle A (2003) Hereditary colorectal cancer. N Engl J Med 348:919-932
12 Santarelli RL, Pierre F, Corpet DE (2008) Processed meat and colorectal cancer: a review of epidemiologic and experimental evidence. Nutr Cancer 60:131-144
13. Kune G, Watson L (2011) Lowering the Risk of Rectal Cancer among Habitual Beer Drinkers by Dietary Means. Adv Prev Med 2011:874048
14. Larsson SC, Wolk A (2007) Obesity and colon and rectal cancer risk: a meta-analysis of prospective studies. Am J Clin Nutr 86:556-565
15. Harriss DJ, Atkinson G, George K et al (2009) Lifestyle factors and colorectal cancer risk (1): systematic review and meta-analysis of associations with body mass index. Colorectal Dis 11:547-563
16. Botteri E, Iodice S, Bagnardi V et al (2008) Smoking and colorectal cancer: a meta-analysis. JAMA 300:2765-2778
17. Paskett ED, Reeves KW, Rohan TE et al (2007) Association between cigarette smoking and colorectal cancer in the Women's Health Initiative. J Natl Cancer Inst 99:1729-1735
18. Cuzick J, Otto F, Baron JA et al (2009) Aspirin and non-steroidal anti-inflammatory drugs for cancer prevention: an international consensus statement. Lancet Oncol 10:501-507

19. Kennedy DA, Stern SJ, Moretti M et al (2011) Folate intake and the risk of colorectal cancer: a systematic review and meta-analysis. Cancer Epidemiol 35:2-10
20. Jaszewski R, Misra S, Tobi M et al (2008) Folic acid supplementation inhibits recurrence of colorectal adenomas: a randomized chemoprevention trial. World J Gastroenterol 14:4492-4498
21. Harriss DJ, Atkinson G, Batterham A et al (2009) Lifestyle factors and colorectal cancer risk (2): a systematic review and meta-analysis of associations with leisure-time physical activity. Colorectal Dis 11:689-701

Pretherapeutic Diagnosis and Staging

2

Emilio Quaia, Luca De Paoli and Maria Assunta Cova

2.1 Introduction

The incidence of colorectal cancer has been rising dramatically following economic development. Currently, colorectal cancer is the third leading cause of cancer deaths in the United States and the second in Europe. Adenocarcinomas comprise the vast majority (98%) of colon and rectal cancers. Other rare rectal cancers include carcinoid (0.4%), lymphoma (1.3%), and sarcoma (0.3%). Squamous cell carcinomas may develop in the transition area from the rectum to the anal verge and are considered anal carcinoma.

Rectal cancer is defined as a malignant tumoral lesion which develops within 16 cm from the anal margin. Rectal cancer presents a higher incidence in males (M/F=2/1) and in the north and west of Europe [1], with a global number of 138,000 new cases per year [2]. Rectal cancer is associated with a poor prognosis because of the risk of both metastases and local recurrence [3]. Histologic variants of rectal adenocarcinoma, such as signet ring, mucinous, medullary, adenosquamous (including glassy cell), undifferentiated, spindle cell, clear cell, hepatoid, and oncocytic, are associated with different clinical outcomes, and almost always with a worse prognosis compared with that of adenocarcinoma at the same disease stage. Mucinous adenocarcinoma is characterized by excess mucin production. It is more aggressive than usual nonvariant adenocarcinomas. Mucinous adenocarcinoma is characterized as affecting younger patients and having a high frequency of lymph node metastases, local recurrence, and advanced stage at presentation.

Total mesorectal excision (TME) is widely accepted as standard surgical

E. Quaia (✉)
Department of Medicine, Surgery and Health Sciences, Radiology Unit,
Cattinara University Hospital,
Trieste, Italy
e-mail: quaia@units.it

N. de Manzini (ed.), *Rectal Cancer,*
Updates in Surgery
DOI: 10.1007/978-88-470-2670-4_2, © Springer-Verlag Italia 2013

practice for rectal cancer [4], and provides the best chance of a tumor-free circumferential resection margin [5]. In TME, the entire mesorectal compartment is removed, including its fascia; this minimizes the chance of tumor being left behind. With this surgical technique, the overall recurrence rate has been reported to be well below 10%, without the help of radiation therapy [6]. Local recurrence is directly related to incomplete resection of the tumor [7, 8] and the most important parameter related to local recurrence is the distance between the tumor and the mesorectal fascia [6, 9]. Locally advanced rectal cancer with extramural spread (T3 tumor) has a high frequency of local recurrence and metastasis. Nowadays, the standard treatment for locally advanced rectal cancer consists of preoperative neoadjuvant concomitant radiation and chemotherapy (CRT) followed by standard resection of the rectum, and resection of the surrounding organs [10, 11].

Nowadays rectal endoscopy is the most accurate diagnostic tool for the preoperative diagnosis of rectal cancer. Preoperative staging and restaging after CRT may be defined by endoluminal ultrasound and magnetic resonance (MR) imaging. There have been many reports on rectal cancer imaging with endorectal ultrasound (US), computed tomography (CT), or magnetic resonance (MR) imaging [3, 12, 13], but most studies focused only on determination of T and N stages rather than on the more important mesorectal fascia.

2.2 The Role of the Different Imaging Techniques in the Staging of Rectal Cancer

2.2.1 Endoluminal Ultrasound

Endoluminal US is an established modality for evaluation of the integrity of the rectal wall layers. Its advantages include convenient accessibility, as in many instances it is part of the initial assessment performed by the colorectal surgeon in conjunction with the digital rectal examination (DRE) [12]. Endoluminal US is performed by using high frequency (>7.5 MHz) endoluminal transducers. The rectal wall is depicted in four layers (excluding the balloon interface) from the hypoechoic mucosa, through the hyperechoic submuscosa, to the hypoechoic muscular layer and the hyperechoic serosal layer. With accuracies for T staging varying between 69% and 97%, endoluminal US is presently the most accurate imaging modality for the assessment of tumor ingrowth into rectal wall layers [13, 14]. In a meta-analysis [15] of 11 studies, sensitivity was shown to be affected by T stage. Endoluminal US is very accurate for staging superficial rectal tumors but is not as useful for staging advanced rectal cancer [16], where the overall staging accuracy is 69%, because the limited depth of acoustic penetration prevents accurate assessment of local tumor extent in bulky T3 and advanced rectal cancers. Although endoluminal US is very accurate in staging superficial rectal cancer, it is less suitable for evaluation of the mesorectal excision plane. Moreover, endoluminal

US is limited in differentiating the T2 from the initial T3 stage [17]. On the other hand, the overall accuracy of endoluminal US in N staging ranges from 64% to 83% [17].

2.2.2 Computed Tomography

In a recently published meta-analysis [18] of 78 studies conducted between 1980 and 1998 in 4,897 patients with rectal cancer, CT showed an accuracy of 73% for T staging. The overall accuracy of N staging ranges from 22% to 80%, considering as metastatic lymph nodes ≥ 1 cm or rounded lymph nodes ≥ 8 mm. The low spatial and contrast resolution of conventional CT protocols does not allow a detailed evaluation of the rectal wall and may have contributed to the low performance of CT for staging superficial tumors. Recent years have seen the development of multidetector CT with sub-millimeter voxel size achievable on modern machines. The high spatial resolution achieved is not accompanied by a similarly high contrast resolution, and it thus remains doubtful whether the high spatial resolution in itself will improve accuracy, since the inherent contrast resolution is poor [12].

2.2.3 Magnetic Resonance Imaging

MR imaging has emerged as the dominant method of pelvic imaging in rectal cancer [19]. The successful introduction of MR imaging for pelvic diseases, due to its superb contrast resolution between tumor and soft tissues, has led to the gradual replacement of CT by MR imaging for local and regional rectal cancer staging. Nowadays superficial phased-array multichannel coils or endoluminal coils are employed.

2.3 MR Imaging – Technical Aspects

In our imaging department the usual MR imaging protocol employed for rectal cancer assessment includes a 1.5-T unit with a minimal gradient intensity of 30 mT/m and a 150 mT/m/msec slew rate, a surface pelvic phased-array coil, and a small field of view. Our usual protocol includes T2-weighted fast spin-echo (TR/TE, 4947/130 ms, turbo factor, 25; slice thickness, 3-4 mm; gap, 0.4 mm; matrix, 512 x 512; voxel dimensions, 0.8 mm^3; field of view, 240-250 mm; acquisitions, 4; total acquisition time, 2 minutes and 23 seconds) MR imaging sequences in the transverse, coronal, and sagittal planes [20]. The axial and coronal oblique images should be obtained orthogonal and parallel to the long axis of the tumor. A 20 mg dose of the intravenous antiperistaltic agent hyoscine-N butylbromide should be administered before starting the MR examination. Gadolinium-enhanced T1-weighted MRI could be omitted in the

MR protocol for preoperative assessment of primary rectal cancer [21]. Recently, we implemented a T1-weighted spectral fat saturation inversion recovery (SPIR) (TR/TE, 598/27 ms; turbo factor, 6; slice thickness, 4 mm; gap, 0.4 mm; matrix, 512 x 512; voxel dimensions, 0,6 mm^3; field of view, 240-250 mm; averages, 2; total acquisition time, 4 minutes and 50 seconds) MR imaging sequence after gadolinium injection (0.1 mmol/kg) to differentiate enhancing tumor infiltration from desmoplastic tissue reaction or reactive fibrosis, after concomitant chemoradiation therapy within the nonenhancing mesorectal fat [22].

2.4 Anatomy of the Rectum for Interpretation of MR Images

The surgical anal canal extends about 3-4 cm, is shorter in women (2-3 cm), and terminates superiorly at the anorectal ring or at the upper portion of the puborectal muscle [19]. The lower limit of the anal canal corresponds to the anal verge and corresponds to the transition between the skin and the anal mucosa [19].

The muscular wall of the anal canal consists of the internal and external sphincter. The internal sphincter represents the continuation of the circular layer of the rectal muscolaris propria while the outer muscular wall is composed by the puborectal muscle and exernal sphincter. The dentate line, corresponding approximately to the upper portion of the external sphincter muscle, is located from 1.5 to 2 cm above the anal verge and is not usually visible on MR imaging, even though it can be ideally located in the lowermost portion of the anal columns.

The rectum extends from the upper limit of the anal canal up to the rectosigmoid junction, with a length of 15 cm. The proximal limit of the rectum is the rectosigmoid junction, 15 cm above the anal verge, while the distal limit corresponds to the anorectal junction at the level of the muscular anorectal ring. On MR imaging, the rectosigmoid junction corresponds to the visceral tract where the rectum is completely covered by the peritoneal layer [19]. The rectum is anatomically divided into three segments: the lower third, middle third, and upper third. The mesorectum consists of the rectum and the surrounding mesorectal or perirectal fat with the perirectal lymph nodes. The mesorectum is covered posteriorly and laterally by a postero-lateral fibrous envelope belonging to the pelvic visceral fascia or mesorectal fascia (MRF), distinct from the parietal pelvic fascia, and anteriorly by the "Denonvilliers' fascia", which covers the posterior surface of the prostate and seminal vesicles in men.

The MRF represents a very important structure to be evaluated in the surgical planning of rectal cancer, particularly if TME is the selected surgical procedure. The MRF can be identified as a thin, low-signal-intensity structure that envelops the mesorectum on MR images. The MRF is more difficult to recognize in the distal and anterior regions of the rectum due to the small amount of fat tissue.

2.5 MRI in the Primary Staging of Rectal Cancer

2.5.1 T-staging

T-staging in rectal cancer is classified as: TX: not determined; T0: no visible tumor; Tis: carcinoma in situ; T1: submucosal tumor only; T2: growth into the muscularis propria; T3: growth into the mesorectal fat; T4: growth into neighbouring organs, or peritoneal infiltration or perforation.

MR imaging or endoscopic ultrasound are the imaging techniques employed to define the T stage of the rectal tumor; they may lead to staging failures in the differentiation of T2 and borderline T3 tumors. Endoluminal US allows a superior image contrast and spatial resolution with a clear depiction of the different layers of the rectal wall [23]. This also allows a more accurate T staging, especially in the differentiation of the T2 and T3 stages with accuracy ranging between 71% and 91% [23, 24]. Endorectal MR imaging has the same accuracy as endorectal US for the staging of superficial tumors[14]. However, the endoluminal coil presents a limited field of view, and the MRF and the surrounding pelvic structures are difficult to visualize owing to the MR signal drop-off at a short distance from the coil. Moreover, the endoluminal coil can be difficult or impossible to insert in patients with rectal stenosis, and failed insertion rates of as high as 40% have been reported in patients with rectal cancer.

Phased-array external coils present a larger field of view and are suitable for the staging of both superficial and advanced rectal tumors [25, 26]. In particular, most staging failures with MR imaging occur in the differentiation of T2-stage and borderline T3-stage lesions (Figs. 2.1, 2.2), with possible understaging (Fig. 2.3) or overstaging. Overstaging is often caused by desmoplastic reactions adjacent to the tumor [27], while it is difficult on MR images to differentiate spiculation in the perirectal fat caused only by fibrosis (stage pT2) from spiculation caused by fibrosis containing tumor cells (stage pT3).

For patients with T3- and/or N1-stage tumors, adjuvant CRT has been the standard in the United States, while neoadjuvant CRT is used in Europe [28]. MR imaging provides an accurate measurement of the depth of extramural tumor spread which makes it possible to put forward a reliable preoperative prognosis (Figs. 2.4, 2.5) [29]. Accurate and detailed anatomic information on tumor extent is essential not only for the selection of patients for neoadjuvant chemotherapy and radiation therapy to achieve tumor shrinkage, but also for planning the optimal surgical procedure.

However, the present T-staging system presents some overt limitations, including the lack of discrimination between tumors distant from the circumferential resection margin (CRM) and tumors close to or with involvement of the CRM [3]. Although most of these tumors are classified as stage T3, they have a different risk of local recurrence. It has been shown that the distance from the rectal tumor to the CRM is the real predictor of the local recurrence rate (see below) [30, 31]. MR imaging should be used to identify tumors that

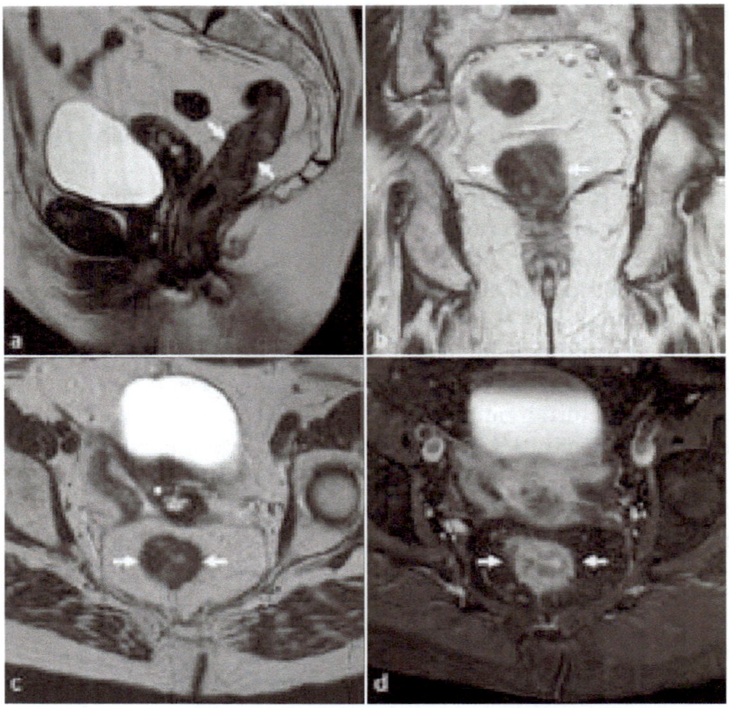

Fig. 2.1 55-year-old woman with a rectal cancer. (**a-d**) Turbo spin-echo T2 weighted sequence (TR/TE, 4947/130) on the longitudinal (**a**), coronal (**b**), and transverse plane (**c**), and spectral presaturation by inversion recovery T1-weighted sequence (TR/TE, 598/27) after gadolinium injection on the transverse plane (**d**). The tumor (*arrows*) is limited to the rectal wall without mesorectal fat infiltration

will have a close or involved CRM so that they can be selected for more extensive (neoadjuvant) treatment.

The major reason for rectal tumor overstaging by MR imaging is diffuse hypointense tissue infiltration into the mesorectal fat [32], due to the difficulty of differentiating reactive fibrosis from residual tumor after neoadjuvant irradiation. Recently, SPIR MR sequence after gadolinium injection was proposed to differentiate enhancing tumor infiltration from desmoplastic tissue reaction or reactive fibrosis after CRT within the nonenhancing mesorectal fat [22].

2.5.2 Locally Advanced Rectal Cancer

Locally advanced rectal cancer has a poor prognosis because of the high frequency of metastasis and local recurrence; a wide surgical resection is needed to remove the tumor with a clear margin. From 10% to 20% of rectal tumors also show infiltration of the surrounding pelvic structures. In these cases, the

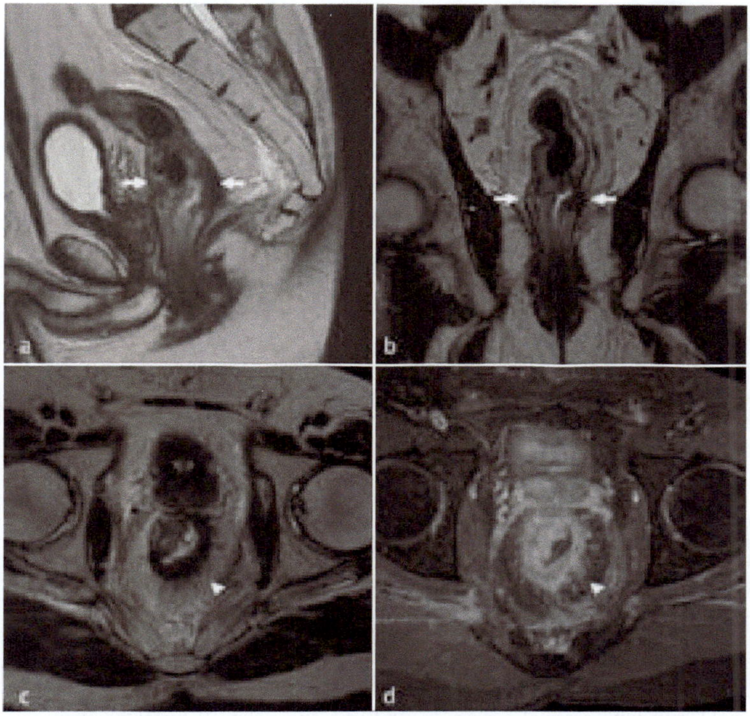

Fig. 2.2 60-year-old man with a rectal cancer treated by radiation therapy with concomitant chemotherapy. (a-d) Turbo spin-echo T2 weighted sequence (TR/TE, 4947/130) on the longitudinal (a), coronal (b), and transverse plane (c), and spectral presaturation by inversion recovery T1-weighted sequence (TR/TE, 598/27) after gadolinium injection on the transverse plane (d). Tumor (*arrow*) with mesorectal fat infiltration. Reticular enhancing strands (*arrowheads*) within the mesorectal fat associated with concomitant enhancing nodules projecting from the rectal wall towards the mesorectal fat

patient's best chance for cure is a radical en bloc resection of the tumor and the surrounding invaded organs [33]. MR imaging was found to be more accurate than CT in the prediction of organ invasion, pelvic wall invasion, and subtle bone marrow invasion [34].

2.5.3 N - staging

For tumors of the upper portion of the rectum, the route of lymphatic spread is upward along the superior vessels to the inferior mesenteric vessels. Tumors of the lower portion of the rectum show an additional lateral lymphatic route along the middle rectal vessels to the internal iliac vessels. In advanced rectal tumors involving the anal canal there may be a downward spread along the inferior rectal vessels to the groin.

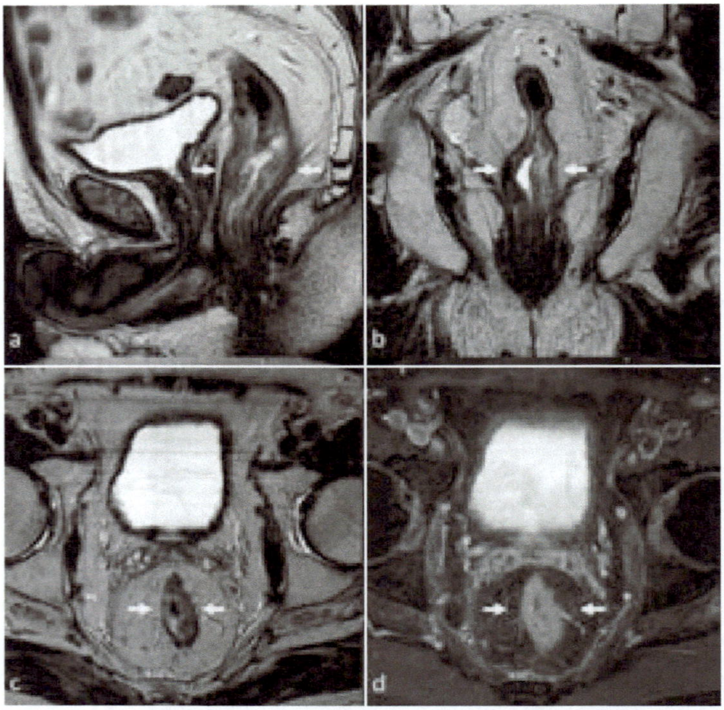

Fig. 2.3 65-year-old man with a rectal cancer. (**a**-**d**) Turbo spin-echo T2 weighted sequence (TR/TE, 4947/130) on the longitudinal (**a**), coronal (**b**), and transverse plane (**c**), and spectral presaturation by inversion recovery T1-weighted sequence (TR/TE, 598/27) after gadolinium injection on the transverse plane (**d**). Tumor (*arrows*) with mesorectal fat infiltration on analysis of the histologic specimen but considered as limited to the rectal wall without mesorectal fat infiltration on MR imaging

Half of the metastatic nodes are within 3 cm of the primary tumor and are smaller than 5 mm in size [35]. With standard TME, the perirectal nodes are removed with the primary tumor, excluding the internal iliac nodes. Since the internal iliac nodes are mainly involved in lower rectal cancer, there is a potential risk that involved internal iliac nodes will be left behind, with the chance of local recurrence. About 28% of lymph node–positive distal rectal cancers have involvement of lateral nodes, and 6% of cases those lateral nodes were the only lymph nodes involved [36]. Some surgeons, mainly from Japan, suggest adding extended pelvic lymphadenectomy to rectal resection. This approach is not favored by most surgeons because of the additional urologic and sexual morbidity, while the benefit is unclear. Probably, a presurgical selection of those patients with the highest risk for lateral lymph node metastases could be useful in centers where pelvic lymphadenectomy is practiced.

The large Dutch TME trial confirmed that nodal disease is a prognostic

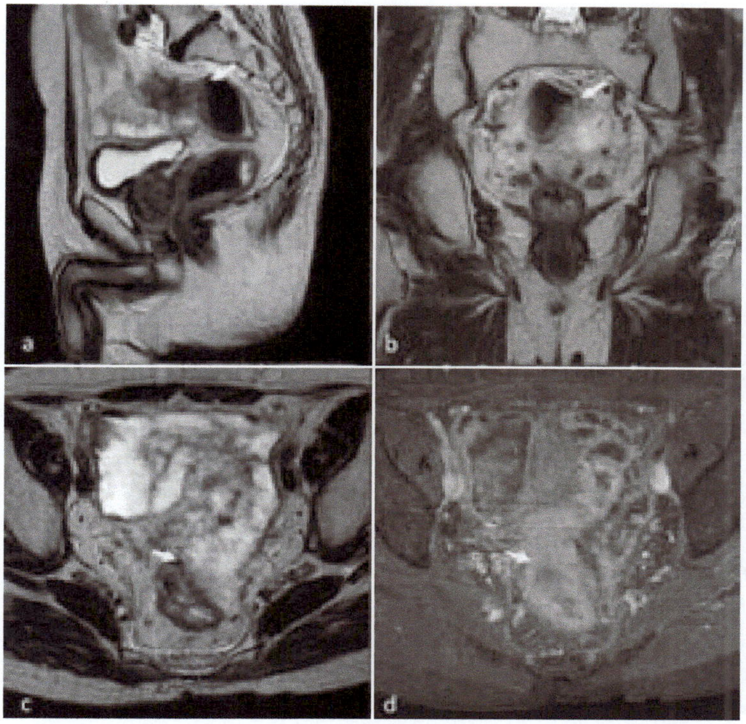

Fig. 2.4 50-year-old man with a rectal cancer treated by radiation therapy with concomitant chemotherapy. (**a-d**) Turbo spin-echo T2 weighted sequence (TR/TE, 4947/130) on the longitudinal (**a**), coronal (**b**), and transverse plane (**c**), and spectral presaturation by inversion recovery T1-weighted sequence (TR/TE, 598/27) after gadolinium injection on the transverse plane (**d**). Tumor with infiltration of the anterior mesorectal fascia and of an ileal loop (*arrows*)

indicator both for distant metastases and local recurrence [11]. In this study, patients with stage III (TxN1) a rectal tumor had a 10-fold higher risk for local recurrence than those with stage I (T1–2N0 stage) tumor, and a threefold higher risk than those with a stage II (T3N0 stage) tumor.

The radiologic assessment of nodal involvement generally relies on morphologic criteria such as the size and shape of the node. However, despite the identification of lymph nodes as small as 2–3 mm on high-spatial-resolution MR images, reliable detection of nodal metastases is presently not possible. Enlarged lymph nodes may be reactive or metastatic, while in small nodes micrometastases are easily missed. In fact, as in other pelvic tumors, rectal cancer is characterized by the high frequency of micrometastases in normal-sized nodes [37]. Large variations in accuracy (62%–83%) for nodal detection can be found for endorectal US [38, 39], as well as for CT (22%–73%) [38, 40]. Accuracy rates for nodal detection with unenhanced MR imaging vary between 39% and 95% [41-43]. Unenhanced MR imaging is not absolutely

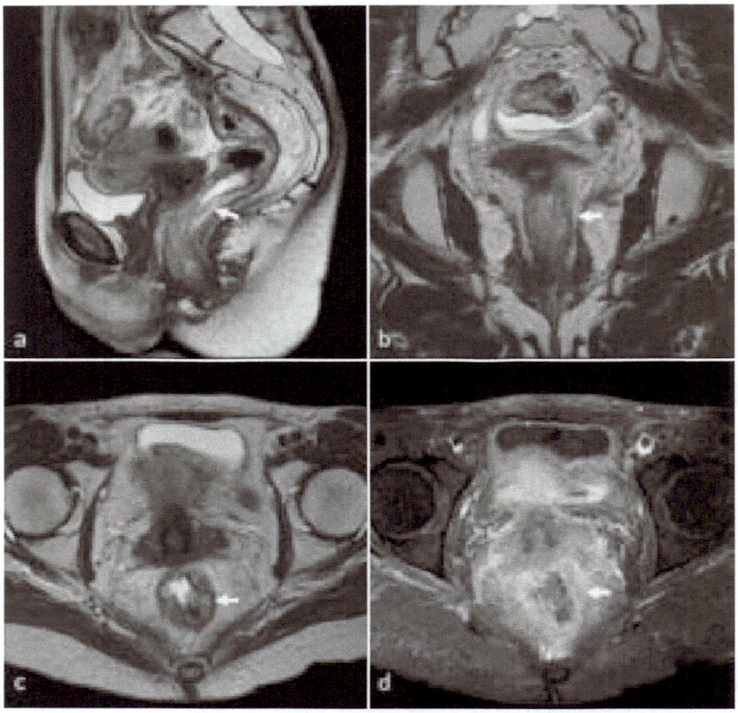

Fig. 2.5 60-year-old man with a rectal cancer treated by radiation therapy with concomitant chemotherapy. (**a**-**d**) Turbo spin-echo T2 weighted sequence (TR/TE, 4947/130) on the longitudinal (**a**), coronal (**b**), and transverse plane (**c**), and spectral presaturation by inversion recovery T1-weighted sequence (TR/TE, 598/27) after gadolinium injection on the transverse plane (**d**). Tumor (*arrow*) with infiltration of visceral peritoneum on the histologic analysis of the tumoral specimen

accurate in distinguishing between inflammatory and metastatic nodes on the basis of signal intensity criteria, even with the use of nonspecific MR contrast agents.

An alternative method would be metabolic imaging by fluorodeoxyglucose positron emission tomography (PET), even though the sensitivity of this method was found to be very low (29%) [44]. The reason for this low sensitivity may be that the proximity of the primary tumor to the urinary bladder obscures small nodal metastases. Recently, high-resolution pelvic MRI has proved more accurate than PET/CT for the prediction of regional nodal status [45].

MR imaging with the use of ultrasmall superparamagnetic iron oxide (USPIO) contrast agents has recently shown promising results for staging nodal metastases. USPIO is a contrast agent that undergoes phagocytosis by the reticuloendothelial system (macrophages in normal lymph nodes). The use of USPIO results in a shortening of the T2* relaxation time and in a decrease in signal intensity on gradient-echo images of normal lymph nodes, owing to increased susceptibility artifacts. These MR properties were used to aid the detection of micrometastases in small lymph nodes. In metastatic nodes, the reticuloendothelial system is displaced by tumor deposits and shows deficits in the uptake of USPIO. Using the pattern of USPIO enhancement had higher diagnostic specificity than, but the same sensitivity as, morphologic findings in pathologically matched mesorectal lymph nodes [46]. Unfortunately, USPIO agents have recently been withdrawn from the market. Recently, gadofosveset-enhanced MR imaging was shown to be an accurate imaging modality for nodal staging and restaging in rectal cancer [47]. Gadofosveset is the first intravascular contrast agent approved for use with magnetic resonance angiography in the European Union. Gadofosveset reversibly binds to albumin, providing extended intravascular enhancement. The metastatic involvement of the node appear as a defect in the uptake of gadofosveset.

2.5.4 Circumferential Resection Margin

According to multiple randomized clinical trials, both preoperative and adjuvant CRT diminish the risk of local recurrence; TME is a surgical technique that removes the rectal tumor and all local draining nodes in an intact package. One of the most important factors determining the success of TME surgery is the relationship of the tumor to the CRM [12]. The measurement of tumor extent relative to the MRF and the prediction of tumor-free CRM on the basis of MR imaging may be more feasible than defining the T stage [27].

Because several studies have shown that neoadjuvant CRT is more efficient and less toxic than postoperative therapy, it has become increasingly important to evaluate the risk of CRM before the operation.

MR imaging is the imaging modality that can most accurately evaluate the risk of tumoral recurrence. The potential CRM or the relationship of the tumor to the MRF has emerged as one of the most powerful predictors of the risk of tumoral recurrence. Surgical dissection outside the MRF has become central in the efforts to achieve CRM negativity and is possible in many cases. In this field terminology is crucial. The term CRM has repeatedly been used in trial protocols, consensus documents, and scientific articles to refer to proximity to the MRF. Preoperatively the most appropriate term is MRF, while postoperatively CRM is the appropriate term [48]. If the MRF is involved or if the tumor extends to a point that is within 1 mm from the MRF, there is a clear risk that CRM will be involved if only a TME is performed. In particularly low rectal tumors, the anal sphincters constitute the corresponding significant border, because the MRF does not extend beyond the puborectal muscle.

Tumor restaging by MR imaging after chemoradiation has moderate accuracy for predicting tumor invasion of the MRF, related to the limitation in differentiating between fibrosis with or without small tumor foci [49].

Adding diffusion-weighted imaging to T2-weighted imaging can improve the prediction of tumor clearance in the MRF after neoadjuvant CRT compared with T2-weighted imaging alone in patients with locally advanced rectal cancer [50].

2.6 MRI after Neoadjuvant Chemoradiation Therapy

Extramural tumor spread influences both long-term survival and the risk of local recurrence in patients with rectal cancer. Locally advanced rectal cancer with extramural spread (T3 tumor) has a high frequency of local recurrence and metastasis. Nowadays, the standard treatment for locally advanced rectal cancer consists of preoperative neoadjuvant CRT followed by standard resection of the rectum, and resection of the surrounding organs that are infiltrated by the rectal tumor [10, 11].

The rationale behind preoperative CRT is first to downstage and downsize locally advanced rectal cancer. Tumor shrinkage due to neoadjuvant CRT is frequently observed (Fig. 2.6), also with pathologically complete responses [51]. The benefits of downstaging and downsizing locally advanced rectal cancer include improvement in resectability, better local control, sphincter preservation, decreased rates of local recurrence, and, most important, improved overall survival.

Radiation therapy is usually performed with a total dose of 5040 cGY over 6 weeks. The radiation field includes the tumor and pelvis. Chemotherapy is usually performed with 425 mg/m2/d of 5-fluorouracil and 20 mg/m2/d of leucovorin during weeks 1 and 5 of radiation therapy, whilesurgical resection is mainly performed 6 weeks after the completion of neoadjuvant CRT. Before

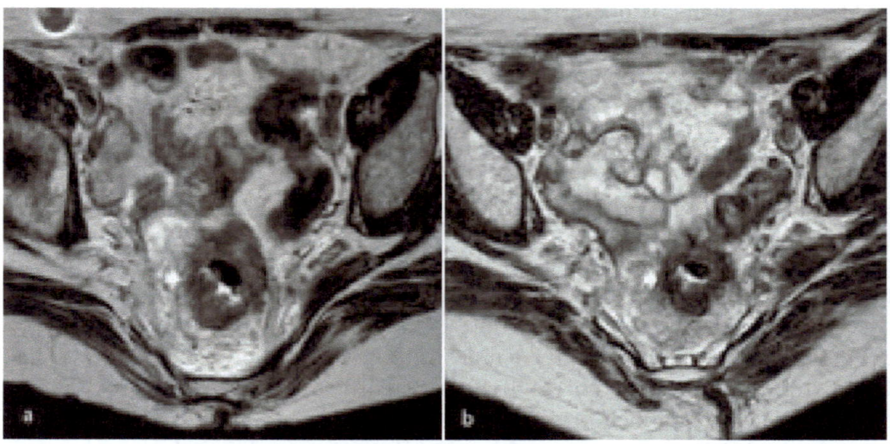

Fig. 2.6 55-year-old man with a rectal cancer before (**a**) and after (**b**) treatment by neoadjuvant radiation therapy with concomitant chemotherapy. Turbo spin-echo T2 weighted sequence (TR/TE, 4947/130) on the transverse plane. Tumor (*arrow*) shows a clear shrinkage after neoadjuvant therapy

the surgery, repeated high-resolution pelvic MR imaging is performed using the same method as for pre-CRT MR imaging.

Imaging studies, especially high-resolution pelvic MR imaging, play a key role in staging rectal cancer before and after CRT. Preliminary results indicate that diffusion-weighted MR imaging, especially at high b values, would be effective for predicting treatment outcome and for early detection of tumor response [51, 52]. In particular, the early increase of mean tumor apparent diffusion coefficient (ADC) and low pretherapy mean ADC in rectal carcinoma correlates with good response to CRT [53, 54].

After CRT, the tumor response is classified as complete response (no residual tumor), partial response (tumor volume decreased > 50% or downstaging), or no response after postoperative pathologic analysis of the tumor specimens. In several studies, CRT has resulted in a 60%–70% tumor response rate, and in particular a 10%–20% complete tumor response rate, leading to improved resectability and local control. Both preoperative and postoperative CRT diminish the risk of local recurrence [55, 56], and the morphologic evaluation and volumetric reduction of the rectal tumor at MR imaging has a strong correlation with response to CRT [57]. Early tumor volume reduction rate after 2 weeks of CRT may be an even better indicator than diffusion-weighted MR imaging based on the mean ADC measurements for predicting CRT treatment outcome [58]. Moreover, post-CRT diffusion-weighted MR volumetry provided high diagnostic performance in assessing complete response and was significantly more accurate than T2-weighted MR volumetry [59].

According to multiple randomized clinical trials in patients with rectal cancer who have received neoadjuvant CRT, MR imaging has an accuracy of 66% in predicting resection margin involvement during restaging of irradiated rectal cancers (sensitivity, 100%; specificity, 35%; positive predictive value, 58%; negative predictive value, 100%) [49]. The reported overall accuracy of MR imaging in predicting the pathologic stage of nonirradiated rectal cancer is 71%–91% (mean, 85%) for T staging, and 43%–85% (75%) for N staging [60-62]. However, the reported overall accuracy of MR imaging in the restaging of irradiated rectal cancer is much lower: 47%–54% (50%) for T staging and 64%–68% (65%) for N staging [10, 49], and is even worse for mucin-producing tumors.

The low accuracy of MR imaging in predicting the pathologic stage of irradiated rectal cancer appears to be related to both overstaging and understaging. The major cause of understaging is nonvisualization of the tumor mass at MR imaging due to viable tumor nets within fibrotic scars in the mesorectal fat. The factors related to overstaging include fibrosis, desmoplastic reaction, edema, and inflammation. CRT reduces the evidence of the peripheral hypointense muscular layer of the rectal wall, and mesorectal fat infiltration becomes difficult to identify. The differentiation of fibrotic scar tissue from tumor infiltration after neoadjuvant CRT is the most important parameter in the prognosis of rectal cancer. Consequently, post-CRT images must be carefully compared with pre-CRT images.

Alterations in the rectum after CRT - such as histopathologic changes in the tumor, or replacement by fibrotic scar tissue with mucin pools [10, 63, 64] - make it difficult to detect viable tumor on unenhanced MR images. This results in a limited accuracy of MR in rectal cancer restaging after CRT. The limited accuracy of MR imaging in predicting mesorectal fat infiltration of non-irradiated rectal cancer is due to the limited capability for differentiation between viable tumor and desmoplastic tissue reaction. In irradiated rectal cancer this limitation is much more important due to the limited capability of MR imaging to differentiate between viable tumor, residual desmoplastic fibrosis, and reactive fibrosis due to scar tissue [52, 57]. This is related to the presence of single or multiple perirectal strands, appearing hypointense on T2-weighted MR images, reaching or not reaching the MRF, which may reflect both tumor infiltration and post-irradiation mesorectal fat fibrosis.

Recent studies of prediction of CRM involvement during restaging of irradiated rectal cancers by using T2-weighted imaging along with gadolium-enhanced T1-weighted imaging demonstrated high diagnostic accuracy (sensitivity, 75%; specificity, 88%–98%; accuracy, 85%–92%; PPV, 66.7%–92.3%; NPV, 91.5%–92.3%) in comparison with that of studies using only T2-weighted imaging (sensitivity, 100%; specificity, 35%; accuracy, 66%; PPV, 58%; NPV, 100%) [61].

Preoperative diagnosis of histologic variants of rectal adenocarcinoma, especially mucinous adenocarcinoma, is important because these variants tend to have a poor response to CRT, and surgical treatment is initially considered. In addition, the excess mucin results in high signal intensity on T2-weighted images, since the lesion retains high signal intensity on T2-weighted images, making it difficult to distinguish between a true mass or remaining mucin.

For lymph node staging, pre-CRT MR imaging has moderate accuracy when size criteria are used. It is difficult to differentiate a metastatic lymph node and irradiated lymph node change with post-CRT MR imaging by using morphologic criteria. In particular, a change in a lymph node with or without metastasis after CRT is assumed to be associated with metastasis, resulting in lymph node overstaging. Some reports have demonstrated the ability of USPIO contrast agents to increase the specificity and accuracy in detecting even small lymph node metastases [65]. Recently, gadofosveset-enhanced MR imaging was shown to be an accurate imaging modality for nodal staging and restaging in rectal cancer [47].

MR volumetry and functional MR imaging may be helpful in the prediction and assessment of tumor response to CRT. Awareness of post-CRT changes helps radiologists achieve appropriate restaging of irradiated rectal cancer with MR imaging, and can lead to a reduction in understaging or overstaging; it is important to obtain and compare both pre- and post-CRT images before interpreting the post-CRT images.

Traditionally, assessment of CRT response with MR imaging was performed with two-dimensional measurements of orthogonal tumor diameters. The disadvantages of this approach are that the measurement is inaccurate owing to the irregular configuration of the colorectal tumor and is not reproducible. Advances in MR imaging techniques and computer technology have led to a reliable calculation of the tumor volume. The volume is reconstructed automatically and calculated by summing each of the cross-sectioned volumes of the entire tumor lesion on the workstation by using software. In comparison with two-dimensional measurement of orthogonal tumor diameters, three-dimensional volume assessment with MR imaging is known to be a highly reliable and objective indicator of actual tumor volume. Before and after CRT, three-dimensional MR volumetry is useful to confirm the downstaging of a tumor in the form of decreased tumor volume, and there is a good correlation between the tumor volume reduction after CRT on MR imaging and histopathologic analysis.

However, MR volumetric evaluation cannot demonstrate any differences between patients with complete histologic regression and those with residual disease.

Dynamic contrast-enhanced MR imaging with tracer kinetic modeling could be useful; it consists in kinetic data analysis after bolus contrast injection with calculation of contrast agent concentration–time courses in tissue, as well as arterial blood. Contrast agent concentrations are inferred from relative signal intensity changes on dynamically acquired MR images. However, this method is prone to errors due to nonlinear signal intensity behavior or tissue-specific influences. The perfusion index (given in milliliters per minute per 100 g), corresponding to the maximum slope of the tissue concentration–time curve divided by the maximum value of the arterial input function, is used to quantify tumor microcirculation, and is measured for each pixel inside the defined tumor region.

The perfusion index is a measure of tissue perfusion and permeability and has been previously used to determine tumor microcirculation. Regression of tumor microcirculation, as shown by using the perfusion index, is considered an important early prognostic factor for treatment response, before reductions in tumor volume. Thus, perfusion MR imaging can be used for prediction of CRT response and for primary tumor staging.

At a high signal intensity, diffusion-weighted MR imaging (diffusion restriction) reflects high cellular density which is suggestive of a malignant lesion. Recent studies have already shown the potential value of high b value diffusion-weighted MR imaging in detection of colorectal cancer [54].

At MR imaging, a high ADC value measured before CRT, reflecting rapid water diffusion into the necrotic area in rectal cancer, is considered a predictor of a poor response to CRT [66]. After CRT, the reduction of tumor cellularity and the increased cell membrane permeability to water molecules determine an increase in water diffusivity and in the ADC, while the increased interstitial fibrosis in previous tumor areas further reduces the restriction of diffusion [52].

References

1. Biondo S, Navarro M, Marti-Rague J et al (2005) Response to neoadjuvant therapy for rectal cancer: influence on long-term results. Colorectal Dis 7:472-479
2. Boyle P, Ferlay J (2005) Cancer incidence and mortality in Europe, 2004. Ann Oncol 16:481-488
3. Beets-Tan R, Beets GL (2004) Rectal cancer: review with emphasis on MR imaging. Radiology 232:335-346
4. Jemal A, Siegel R, Ward E et al (2007) Cancer statistics 2007. CA Cancer J Clin 57:43-66
5. Nagtegaal ID, Gosens M (2007) Combinations of tumor and treatment parameters are more discriminative for prognosis than the present TNM system in rectal cancer. J Clin Oncol 25:1647-1650
6. Heald RJ, Ryall RDH (1986) Recurrence and survival after total mesorectal excision for rectal cancer. Lancet 1:1479-1482
7. Adam IJ, Mohamdee MO, Martin IG et al (1994) Role of circumferential margin involvement in the local recurrence of rectal cancer. Lancet 344:707-711
8. Quirke P, Durdey P, Dixon MF, Williams NS (1986) Local recurrence of rectal adenocarcinoma due to inadequate surgical resection: histopathological study of lateral tumor spread and surgical excision. Lancet 2:996-999
9. Reynolds JV, Joyce WP, Dolan J et al (1996) Pathological evidence in support of total mesorectal excision in the management of rectal cancer. Br J Surg 83:1112-1115
10. Allen SD, Padhani AR, Dzik-Jurasz AS, Glynne-Jones R (2007) Rectal carcinoma: MRI with histologic correlation before and after chemoradiation therapy. AJR Am J Roentgenol 188:442-451
11. Kapiteijn E, Marijnen CAM, Nagtegaal ID et al (2001) Preoperative radiotherapy combined with total mesorectal excision for resectable rectal cancer. N Engl J Med 345:638-646
12. Brown G, Daniels I (2005) Preoperative Staging of Rectal Cancer: The MERCURY Research Project. Recent Results in Cancer Research 165:58-74
13. Rifkin MD, Ehrlich SM, Marks G (1989). Staging of rectal carcinoma: prospective comparison of endorectal US and CT. Radiology 170:319-322
14. Maldjian C, Smith R, Kilger A et al (2000) Endorectal surface coil MR imaging as a staging technique for rectal carcinoma: a comparison study to rectal endosonography. Abdom Imaging 25:75-80
15. Solomon MJ, McLeod RS (1993) Endoluminal transrectal ultrasonography: accuracy, reliability, and validity. Dis Colon Rectum 36:200-205
16. Garcia-Aguilar J, Pollack J, Lee SH et al (2002) Accuracy of endorectal ultrasonography in preoperative staging of rectal tumors. Dis Colon Rectum 45:10-15
17. Schaffzin DM, Wong WD (2004) Endorectal ultrasound in the preoperative evaluation of rectal cancer. Clin Colorectal Cancer 4:124-132
18. Kwok H, Bissett IP, Hill GL (2000) Preoperative staging of rectal cancer. Int J Colorectal Dis 15:9-20
19. Torkzad MR, Påhlman L, Glimelius B (2010) Magnetic resonance imaging (MRI) in rectal cancer: a comprehensive review. Insights Imaging 1:245-267
20. MERCURY Study Group (2006) Diagnostic accuracy of preoperative magnetic resonance imaging in predicting curative resection of rectal cancer: prospective observational study. BMJ 333:779-785
21. Jao SY, Yang BY, Weng HH et al (2010) Evaluation of gadolinium-enhanced T1-weighted magnetic resonance imaging in the preoperative assessment of local staging in rectal cancer. Colorectal Dis 12:1139-1148
22. Quaia E, Ulcigrai V, Coss M et al (2011) Spectral Presaturation Inversion-Recovery MR Imaging Sequence after Gadolinium Injection to Differentiate Fibrotic Scar Tissue and Neoplastic Strands in the Mesorectal Fat in Patients Undergoing Restaging of Rectal Carcinoma after Neoadjuvant Chemo- and Radiation Therapy. Acad Radiol 18:1365-1375
23. Vogl TJ, Pegios W, Mack MG et al (1997) Accuracy of staging rectal tumors with contrast-enhanced transrectal MR imaging. AJR Am J Roentgenol 168:1427-1434

24. Zagoria RJ, Schlarb CA, Ott DJ et al (1997) Assessment of rectal tumor infiltration utilizing endorectal MR imaging and comparison with endoscopic rectal sonography. J Surg Oncol 64:312-317
25. Blomqvist L, Machado M, Rubio C et al (2000) Rectal tumor staging: MR imaging using pelvic phased-array and endorectal coils vs endoscopic ultrasonography. Eur Radiol 10:653-660
26. Hadfield MB, Nicholson AA, MacDonald AW et al (1997) Preoperative staging of rectal carcinoma by magnetic resonance imaging with a pelvic phased-array coil. Br J Surg 84:529-531
27. Beets-Tan RG, Beets GL, Vliegen RF et al (2001) Accuracy of magnetic resonance imaging in prediction of tumor-free resection margin in rectal cancer surgery. Lancet 357:497-504
28. Minsky BD (2001) Adjuvant radiation therapy for rectal cancer: is there finally an answer? (editorial). Lancet 358:1285-1286
29. MERCURY Study Group (2007) Extramural Depth of Tumor Invasion at Thin-Section MR in Patients with Rectal Cancer: Results of the MERCURY Study. Radiology 243:132-139
30. Nagtegaal ID, Marijnen CA, Kranenbarg EK et al (2002) Circumferential margin involvement is still an important predictor of local recurrence in rectal carcinoma: not one millimeter but two millimeters is the limit. Am J Surg Pathol 26:350-357
31. Wibe A, Rendedal PR, Svensson E et al (2002) Prognostic significance of the circumferential resection margin following total mesorectal excision for rectal cancer. Br J Surg 89:327-334
32. Dresen RC, Beets GL, Rutten HJ et al (2009) Locally advanced rectal cancer: MR imaging for restaging after neoadjuvant radiation therapy with concomitant chemotherapy. Part I. Are we able to predict tumor confined to the rectal wall? Radiology 252:71-80
33. Poeze M, Houbiers JG, van de Velde CJ et al (1995) Radical resection of locally advanced colorectal cancer. Br J Surg 82:1386-1390
34. Beets-Tan RG, Beets GL, Borstlap AC et al (2000) Preoperative assessment of local tumor extent in advanced rectal cancer: CT or high-resolution MRI? Abdom Imaging 25:533-541
35. Monig SP, Baldus SE, Zirbes TK et al (1999) Lymph node size and metastatic infiltration in colon cancer. Ann Surg Oncol 6:579-581
36. Moriya Y, Sugihara K, Akasu T, Fujita S (1997) Importance of extended lymphadenectomy with lateral node dissection for advanced lower rectal cancer. World J Surg 21:728-732
37. Bjelovic M, Kalezic V, Petrovic M et al (1998) Correlation of macroscopic and histological characteristics in the regional lymph nodes of patients with rectal and sigmoidal adenocarcinoma. Hepatogastroenterology 45:433-438
38. Beynon J, Mortensen NJ, Foy DM et al (1989) Preoperative assessment of mesorectal lymph node involvement in rectal cancer. Br J Surg76:276-279
39. Tio TL, Coene PP, van Delden OM, Tytgat GN (1991) Colorectal carcinoma: preoperative TNM classification with endosonography. Radiology 179:165-170
40. Balthazar EJ, Megibow AJ, Hulnick D, Naidich DP (1988) Carcinoma of the colon: detection and preoperative staging by CT0. AJR Am J Roentgenol 150:301-306
41. de Lange EE, Fechner RE, Edge SB, Spaulding CA (1990) Preoperative staging of rectal carcinoma with MR imaging: surgical and histopathologic correlation. Radiology 176:623-628
42. McNicholas MM, Joyce WP, Dolan J et al (1994) Magnetic resonance imaging of rectal carcinoma: a prospective study. Br J Surg 81:911-914
43. Thaler W, Watzka S, Martin F et al (1994) Preoperative staging of rectal cancer by endoluminal ultrasound vs.magnetic resonance imaging: preliminary results of a prospective, comparative study. Dis Colon Rectum 37:1189-1193
44. Abdel-Nabi H, Doerr RJ, Lamonica DM et al (1998) Staging of primary colorectal carcinomas with fluorine-18 fluorodeoxyglucose whole-body PET: correlation with histopathologic and CT findings. Radiology 206:755-760
45. Kim DJ, Kim JH, Ryu YH et al (2011) Nodal Staging of Rectal Cancer: High-Resolution Pelvic MRI Versus 18F-FDGPET/CT. J Comput Assist Tomogr 35:531-534
46. Koh DM, George C, Temple L et al (2010) Diagnostic accuracy of nodal enhancement pattern of rectal cancer at MRI enhanced with ultrasmall superparamagnetic iron oxide: findings in pathologically matched mesorectal lymph nodes. AJR Am J Roentgenol 194:505-513

47. Lambregts DM, Beets GL, Maas M et al (2011) Accuracy of gadofosveset-enhanced MRI for nodal staging and restaging in rectal cancer. Ann Surg 253:539-545
48. Glimelius B, Beets-Tan R, Blomqvist L et al (2011) Mesorectal fascia instead of circumferential resection margin in preoperative staging of rectal cancer. J Clin Oncol 29:2142-2143
49. Vliegen RF, Beets GL, Lammering G et al (2008) Mesorectal fascia invasion after neoadjuvant chemotherapy and radiation therapy for locally advanced rectal cancer: accuracy of MR imaging for prediction. Radiology 246:454-462
50. Park MJ, Kim SH, Lee SJ, Jang KM et al (2011) Locally advanced rectal cancer: added value of diffusion-weighted MR imaging for predicting tumor clearance of the mesorectal fascia after neoadjuvant chemotherapy and radiation therapy. Radiology 260:771-780
51. Barbaro B, Vitale R, Leccisotti L et al (2010) Restaging locally advanced rectal cancer with MR imaging after chemoradiation therapy. Radiographics 30:699-716
52. Kim DJ, Kim JH, Lim JS et al (2010) Restaging of rectal cancer with MR imaging after concurrent chemotherapy and radiation therapy. Radiographics 30:503-516
53. Kim SH, Lee JM, Hong SH et al (2009) Locally advanced rectal cancer: added value of diffusion-weighted MR imaging in the evaluation of tumor response to neoadjuvant chemo- and radiation therapy. Radiology 253:116-125
54. Sun YS, Zhang XP, Tang L et al (2010) Locally advanced rectal carcinoma treated with preoperative chemotherapy and radiation therapy: preliminary analysis of diffusion-weighted MR imaging for early detection of tumor histopathologic downstaging. Radiology 254:170-178
55. Glimelius B, Grönberg H, Järhult J et al (2003) A systemic overview of radiation therapy effects in rectal cancer. Acta Oncol 42:476-492
56. Glimelius B, Holm T, Blomquist L (2008) Chemotherapy in addition to preoperative radiotherapy in locally advanced rectal cancer: A systematic overview. Rev Recent Clin Trials 3:204-211
57. Barbaro B, Fiorucci C, Tebala C et al (2009) Locally advanced rectal cancer: MR imaging in prediction of response after preoperative chemotherapy and radiation therapy. Radiology 250:730-739
58. Kim YC, Lim JS, Keum KC et al (2011) Comparison of diffusion-weighted mri and mr volumetry in the evaluation of early treatment outcomes after preoperative chemoradiotherapy for locally advanced rectal cancer. J Magn Reson Imaging 34:570-576
59. Curvo-Semedo L, Lambregts DM, Maas M et al (2011) Rectal cancer: assessment of complete response to preoperative combined radiation therapy with chemotherapy—conventional MR volumetry versus diffusion-weighted MR imaging. Radiology 260:734-743
60. Kuo LJ, Chern MC, Tsou MH et al (2005) Interpretation of magnetic resonance imaging for locally advanced rectal carcinoma after preoperative chemoradiation therapy. Dis Colon Rectum 48:23-28
61. Chen CC, Lee RC, Lin JK et (2005) How accurate is magnetic resonance imaging in restaging rectal cancer in patients receiving preoperative combined chemoradiotherapy? Dis Colon Rectum 48:722-728
62. Reerink O, Verschueren RC, Szabo BG et al (2003) A favourable pathological stage af¬ter neoadjuvant radiochemotherapy in patients with initially irresectable rectal cancer correlates with a favourable prognosis. Eur J Cancer 39:192-195
63. Dworak O, Keilholz L, Hoffmann A (1997) Pathological features of rectal cancer after preoperative radiochemotherapy. Int J Colorectal Dis 12:19-23
64. Torkzad MR, Lindholm J, Martling A et al (2007) MRI after preoperative radiotherapy for rectal cancer; correlation with histopathology and the role of volumetry. Eur Radiol 17:1566-1573
65. Lahaye MJ, Engelen SM, Kessels AG et al (2008) USPIO-enhanced MR imaging for nodal staging in patients with primary rectal cancer. Predictive criteria. Radiology 246:804-811
66. Roth Y, Tichler T, Kostenich G et al (2004) High-b-Value Diffusion-weighted MR Imaging for Pretreatment Prediction and Early Monitoring of Tumor Response to Therapy in Mice. Radiology 686:685-692

Pathology

3

Fabrizio Zanconati, Alessandro De Pellegrin
and Andrea Romano

3.1 Introduction

The anatomical peculiarities of the rectum justify the care that pathologists must take in handling the surgical specimen, because of the rectum's extraperitoneal topography, along with scientific evidence that indicates fascial resection margin (or circumferential margin) [1] and nodal status as major factors impacting on the risk of relapse.

In addition, new possibilities of treatment (neoadjuvant combined complementary therapy and transanal microsurgery) require a multidisciplinary assessment for each patient. Only if all the professionals involved in patient care work together to exchange expertise and knowledge can excellence in quality of care be achieved.

3.2 Role of the Surgeon

The surgical specimen should be submitted to the Anatomic Pathology Laboratory intact as surgically removed, either without fixative (within 1 hour of devascularization) or in appropriate containers with a suitable quantity of buffered formalin (the ideal ratio between specimen weight and formalin volume should be at least equal to 1:2).

The specimen must be accompanied by a request form completely filled in with all the patient's records. However, to allow the pathologist to make a correct and complete diagnosis, the following clinical data must always be included:

F. Zanconati (✉)
Department of Medicine, Surgery and Health Sciences, Pathology Unit,
Cattinara University Hospital,
Trieste, Italy
e-mail: fabrizio.zanconati@aots.sanita.fvg.it

N. de Manzini (ed.), *Rectal Cancer*,
Updates in Surgery
DOI: 10.1007/978-88-470-2670-4_3,

1. the most important data to be communicated to the pathology laboratory is what if any neoadjuvant treatment has been given to the patient (it is also useful to specify the type, dosage and date of the end of treatment);
2. clinical staging: particularly pre- and post- neoadjuvant therapy CT and/or MR staging (preferably including medical report);
3. any difficulties during surgery (attach a schematic diagram to facilitate recognition of the topography and help the pathologist in subsequent sampling);
4. any anamnesis of correlated clinical conditions: inflammatory bowel disease (IBD); familial adenomatous polyposis (FAP) and hereditary nonpolyposis syndrome (HNPCC);
5. date and results of any preoperative diagnostic biopsy performed.

3.3 Role of the Pathologist (Grossing Phase)

The description below refers to colorectal resections and abdominoperineal (Miles) amputations for rectal carcinomas.

Macroscopic examination is of extreme importance for the correct selection of definitive histological specimens, and has been shown to be essential for a correct prognostic stratification of the patient and as an external quality control for assessing surgical procedures. This phase, once considered a marginal part of the pathologist's work, is now an essential instrument for interdisciplinary auditing. The guidelines accepted in Europe by the Consensus Conference EURECA-CC2 of 2009 [2] on the handling of surgical specimens are those proposed by the Royal College of Pathologists (RCP) [3].

When the pathologist has evaluated all the documents available (preferably enclosed with the request), the surgical specimen is measured and its external appearance assessed to evaluate the integrity of the nonperitonealized resection margin (complete, partial or incomplete), the surgical resection plane (mesorectal, intramesorectal or muscular), and the presence or absence of any perforations (spontaneous or iatrogenic) (Fig. 3.1).

In the next step, before any other handling, the non-peritonealized resection margin is carefully inked; the specimen is then opened with an enterotome, starting from the proximal end and proceeding along the antimesenteric side of the bowel (following the line defined by the tenia coli). Extreme care must be taken in determining the position of the neoplasia (particularly if there has been prior neoadjuvant therapy)*. Before the specimen is completely opened, the lumen in the proximity of the tumor should be explored

*It is strongly recommended that, in the diagnostic phase, the endoscope operator should mark the external perimeter of the lesion with biomarker, to make it easy to detect the neoplastic area in the event of a complete post-therapy tumor regression and facilitate sampling.

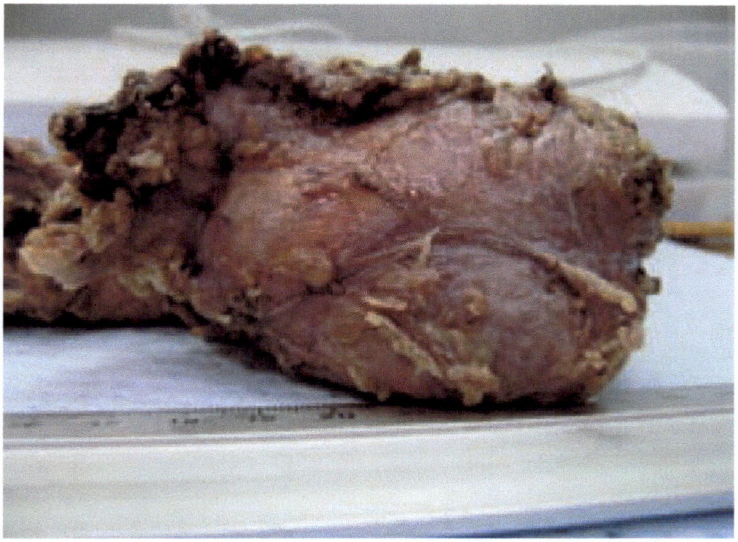

Fig. 3.1 Optimal surgical specimen with complete CRM without incisions or breaks

digitally to exclude any circumferential extension of the lesion; if the lesion does not extend circumferentially, the bowel can be completely opened, respecting the integrity of the lesion. The best way to fix the specimen correctly is to stretch it, pinning it on a cork board (at least the part corresponding to the lesion) and leaving it to fix for 24 hours. The sample is then removed from the support, the formalin replaced, and fixation extended for a further 24 hours.

If the neoplasia involves the whole circumference wall, stop the opening process, insert sponges or tissue paper at the level of the unopened portion and put the whole sample in buffered formalin for 24 hours. It is advisable to extend the fixation for a further 24 hours and then directly perform circumferential serial sections of the bowel.

In both cases the overall fixation time must not be less than 48 hours.

On completion of the fixation phase, the lesion is measured (Fig. 3.2) and its macroscopic appearance described (vegetating, ulcerative, stenosing, linitis plastica-like); the distance from all the resection margins (distal, proximal, including the distance from the peritoneal reflection) is also measured.

In the case of noncircumferential lesions, it is important to indicate the topographical location of the lesion (anterior, posterior, right or left side).

Continue with serial sections orthogonal to the longest axis extending through the entire wall (nonperitonealized margin and/or serosa and mesorectal lymph nodes), including the whole lesion up to 2 cm up- and downstream of its macroscopic limit. On completing this phase, measure the minimum

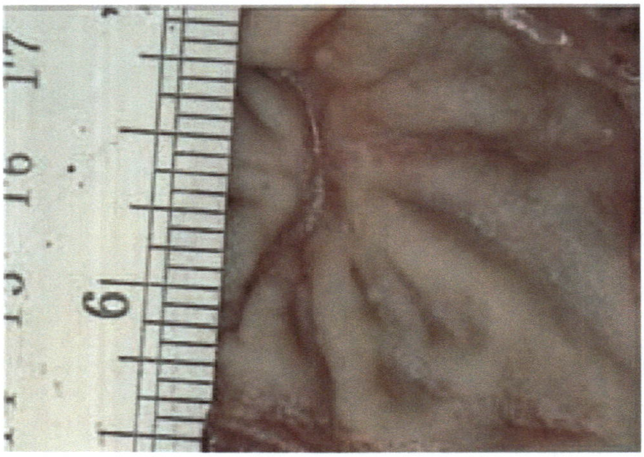

Fig. 3.2 Residual ulcerated lesion after neoadjuvant therapy

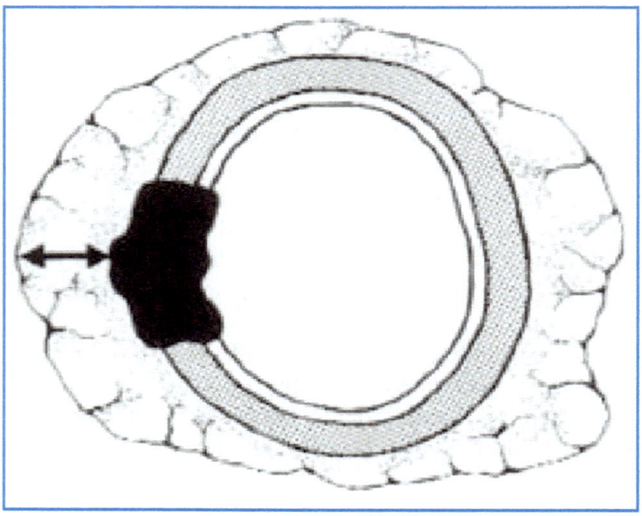

Fig. 3.3 Minimum distance between lesion and CRM (diagram)

macroscopic distance of the lesion from the nonperitonealized resection margin (Figs. 3.3, 3.4, 3.5).

Finally, describe any additional lesions found (polyps, diverticula, ischemic areas, adherence to the viscera, etc).

Each phase should be accompanied by photographs showing:

- quality of the nonperitonealized resection margin;
- appearance of the lesion;

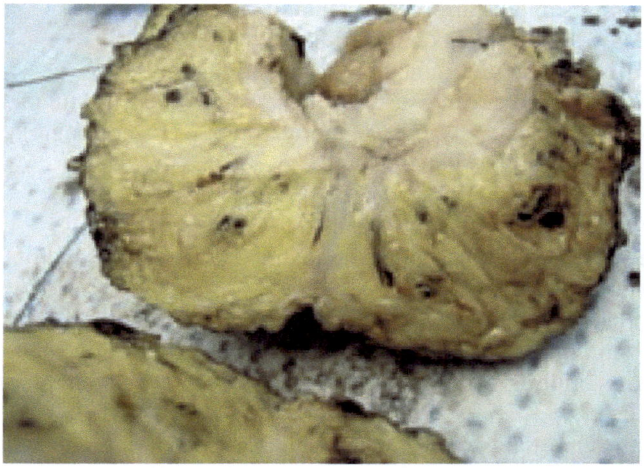

Fig. 3.4 Fibrous striae projecting into mesorectal fat. This patient had been assessed as ycT3 by MRI performed after neoadjuvant therapy. Microscopic examination showed the presence of regression-like fibrous streaks in the absence of viable neoplastic elements

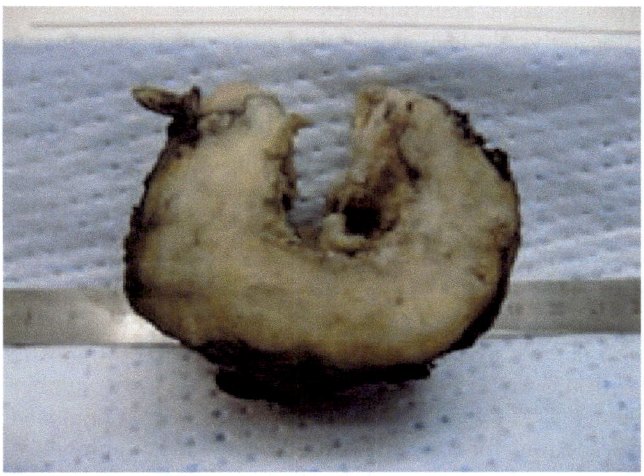

Fig. 3.5 CRM macroscopically involved in the neoplastic process

- topographic relations to any adherent viscera;
- images including all the serial sections, with high magnification of the maximum point of macroscopic infiltration; they should especially document any fibrous striae in the perirectal fat. These images, in our opinion, are extremely useful for subsequent microscopic assessment, and particularly in the case of neoadjuvant therapy, for correlation with MRI and preoperative clinical staging [4].

The following minimum samples are recommended:

- at least four samples of the tumor to demonstrate:
  - the maximum infiltration of the tumor in the intestinal wall;
  - any involvement of the serosa (the surface of the serosa near the tumor should always be inked, especially if it is bumpy, rough or hemorrhagic);
  - the invasion of extramural vascular structures;
  - the relation of the neoplasia with normal-appearing mucosa;
  - the possible involvement of adjacent organs.
- at least one sample representing the nonperitonealized "critical" resection margin in correspondence to the lesion;
- if the lesion is less than 30 mm from the proximal or distal resection margin (rectal or anal), an appropriate section of the "critical" resection margin is required. Total sampling of the resection ring of the surgical stapler should be performed:
  - the resection margins must always be documented in the event of preoperatory diagnosis of undifferentiated lesions or signet ring cell carcinomas, even if the macroscopic limit of the lesion is over 30 mm from the margin;
- a sample of macroscopically intact intestinal wall;
- any other lesions or macroscopic abnormalities:
  - in particular, all the polypoid lesions should be described in terms of dimensions and distance either from the nearest margin or from the main lesion, and suitably documented in the sampling phase.

Lymph node sampling deserves a separate mention because it is one of the most critical phases and has the greatest impact on the subsequent therapeutic course of the patient. It has now been established in literature that the total number of lymph nodes found is an essential parameter for the correct stratification of the risk of progression; in fact, both in the sixth and the current edition of its Staging Manual [5], the AJCC, suggests isolating at least 12 lymph nodes in an adequate surgical specimen. This recommendation derives from the observation in several centres that stages I and II include two prognostic sub-groups; the group with the worse prognosis is the one with a low number of total lymph nodes detected. A recent observational study which analysed more than 80,000 colon resections for cancer showed how the mean number of lymph nodes found for each case has increased, but this has not been followed by an increase of high-stage cases [6].

However, our experience, although agreeing with what has been proposed by the RCP, suggests that it is not advisable to stop when the minimum number of lymph nodes is reached: the gold standard for the pathologist in the sampling phase should be to find all the macroscopically recognisable nodes. It has been highlighted that the problem of the total number of lymph nodes not only has a significant effect on III-II downstaging, but represents a further instrument for risk stratification. Indeed, as has been described for gastric carcinoma [7], and for gastrointestinal carcinomas in general, the relation between positive lymph nodes and total lymph nodes found is an independent risk factor for global and disease-free survival [8, 9].

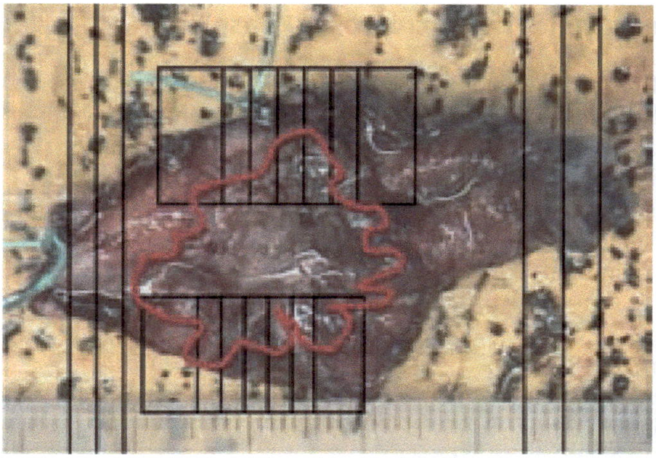

Fig. 3.6 Technique for sampling microsurgical specimen

The sections where the lesion is located may already include appropriately documented lymph nodes with non-peritonealized resection margins; the pathologist's job is to scrupulously investigate the remaining adipous perivisceral tissue, searching for further possible nodules attributable to lymph nodes, distinguishing the mesorectal from the mesocolic nodes and possibly putting the apical nodule (located in proximity to the main vascular ligature in correspondence to the lower mesenteric vessels) into a separate specimen cassette. In some cases, especially after neoadjuvant therapy, the search for lymph nodes is extremely challenging and frustrating, and often the first investigation does not even reach the minimum objective. Whether neoadjuvant therapy has been given or not, and only when the first search has proved unsatisfactory, the recommendation in these cases is to put the adipous perivisceral tissue into clarifying liquid (Carnoy's solution, acetone, Bouin liquid) for 24 hours and carry out a second search for any residual lymph nodes [10].

The following part describes the handling of specimens obtained by transanal microsurgery.

The specimen must be submitted to the pathologist laid out and pinned to a cork board (or similar); at least two anatomical landmarks should be indicated.

The pathologist measures the specimen and describes and measures the lesion; the specimen will then be inked and sectioned, respecting the surgical landmarks. The sampling must be modulated according to the characteristics of the specimen, and especially to the relation between the lesion and resection margins. If the sectioning of one of the margins does not allow this relation to be assessed correctly, a wide section orthogonal to the long axis should be performed; it will also be useful subsequently to perform sections perpendicular to the previous one, including the whole margin with serial parallel sections (Fig. 3.6).

3.4 Role of the Pathologist (Microscopic Phase)

The accuracy of the final pathological report will depend on the accuracy of the pre-analytical and macroscopic phases. The more precise and reliable they are, the more accurate and complete the final report will be. The need for scientific evidence requires pathologists to add to the report not only the histotype but also other histoprognostic parameters that may help in stratifying the risk of progression of the disease.

Accordingly, as a minimum requirement, the report must describe the following features:

- histotype:
  - adenocarcinoma, NAS
  - mucinous adenocarcinoma
  - signet ring cell carcinoma
  - squamous/adenosquamous carcinoma
  - medullary carcinoma
  - undifferentiated carcinoma
  - neuroendocrine neoplasms
  - other
- grading (according to the WHO): assessed on the basis of the percentage of neoplasms forming well-recognizable glands. It is well known that large lesions especially have different degrees of differentiation, so the main and the less differentiated patterns must be pointed out in the report, ensuring that the worst one is highlighted in the final epicrisis.

  The report should also contain further prognostic parameters:
- infiltration pattern: it should be defined whether the lesion's growth pattern is expansive with pushing margins, or infiltrative with intramural finger-like projections;
- desmoplasia: the extent of intra- and perilesional fibrous reaction must be defined; if present, this factor seems to be correlated to a better prognosis [11]. In patients treated with neoadjuvant radiotherapy, the desmoplastic reaction may be an effect of the therapy itself rather than a neoplastic feature [12];
- necrosis: the necrosis rate is graded by trying to exclude the common "dirty" intraglandular necrosis from true tumor necrosis;
- inflammatory cells: the amount of the perilesional lymphocyte cells should be graded (on the periphery of the invasion border);
- angioinvasion: the presence or absence of features suggesting lymphatic or hematic angioinvasion must be defined along with the site (intramural and/or extramural). The seventh edition of TNM suggests not specifying the type of vessels involved (lymphatic vs. hematic, often difficult to distinguish on histological sections), but only LVI (Lympho-Vascular Invasion) will be reported in the epicrisis;
- another important element, assessed as an independent risk factor of lymph node involvement [13] and of recurrence [14] (especially in patients treat-

ed with neoadjuvant therapy [15]) is the presence of perineural sheath infiltration;

- some pathologists evaluate the extent of tumoral budding (isolated neoplastic elements beyond the growth border of the tumoral lesion [16]) in surgical specimens as well as in degenerated polyps [17, 18], but as yet there is no significant evidence of the clinical utility of this additional information.

In the case of lesions treated with neoadjuvant therapy, it is essential to assess the extent of the tumor regression, which can be evaluated on the basis of the presence of microcalcifications, fibrous streaks, giant cells, acellular mucin lakes, etc. Different classification methods have been proposed to assess the degree of response to the neoadjuvant therapy, but currently there is still no shared consensus as to which classification has the greatest impact on the prognosis [19]. The main classifications used are:

- Mandard classification: Mandard's original work assessed the response to neoadjuvant therapy of carcinomas of the oesophagus; only subsequently was this classification introduced for rectal carcinoma [20];
- Dworak classification [21];
- CAP (College of American Pathologists) classification system;
- RCP (Royal College of Pathologists) classification system.

As these classifications have all demonstrated good inter- and intraobserver reproducibility, they may be regarded as having equal validity. In the absence of consensus, the choice of one or the other should be left to the pathologist, who must, however, specify the classification used to avoid a wrong interpretation by the clinician (e.g. for Mandard: 0= complete pathological response, for Dworak: 0= absence of response) (Fig. 3.7).

For staging, the AJCC manual, 2010 edition [5] (Table 3.1) must be used. The staging of cases subjected to neoadjuvant therapy is preceded (in accordance with the AJCC indications) by the prefix y; cases with complete pathological response (absence of residual neoplasia on histological specimens) must be staged as ypT0.

Since a pT staging, pre-neoadjuvant therapy is not by definition possible, the extent of the response should be gathered from the correlation with the clinical staging (TC and/or MRI), pre- vs. post-neoadjuvant therapy (cT vs. ycT), the latter integrated with what was determined by the final pathological staging performed on the surgical specimen (see Fig. 3.4).

The literature indicates that with the same N and M, the pT3 stage has a different stratification of risk of progression in relation to the depth of invasion beyond the muscolaris propria [22]; a pT3 substaging (a,b,c,d) has consequently been proposed that includes the measurement in millimetres of the extension of the neoplasia beyond the muscolaris propria [23].

The epicrisis of the pathological report should always specify not only any involvement of the proximal or distal margins (suffix R of the AJCC), but also the involvement or not of the non-peritonealized resection margin (CRM: Circumferential Resection Margin or MRF: MesoRectal Fascia [24]), indicat-

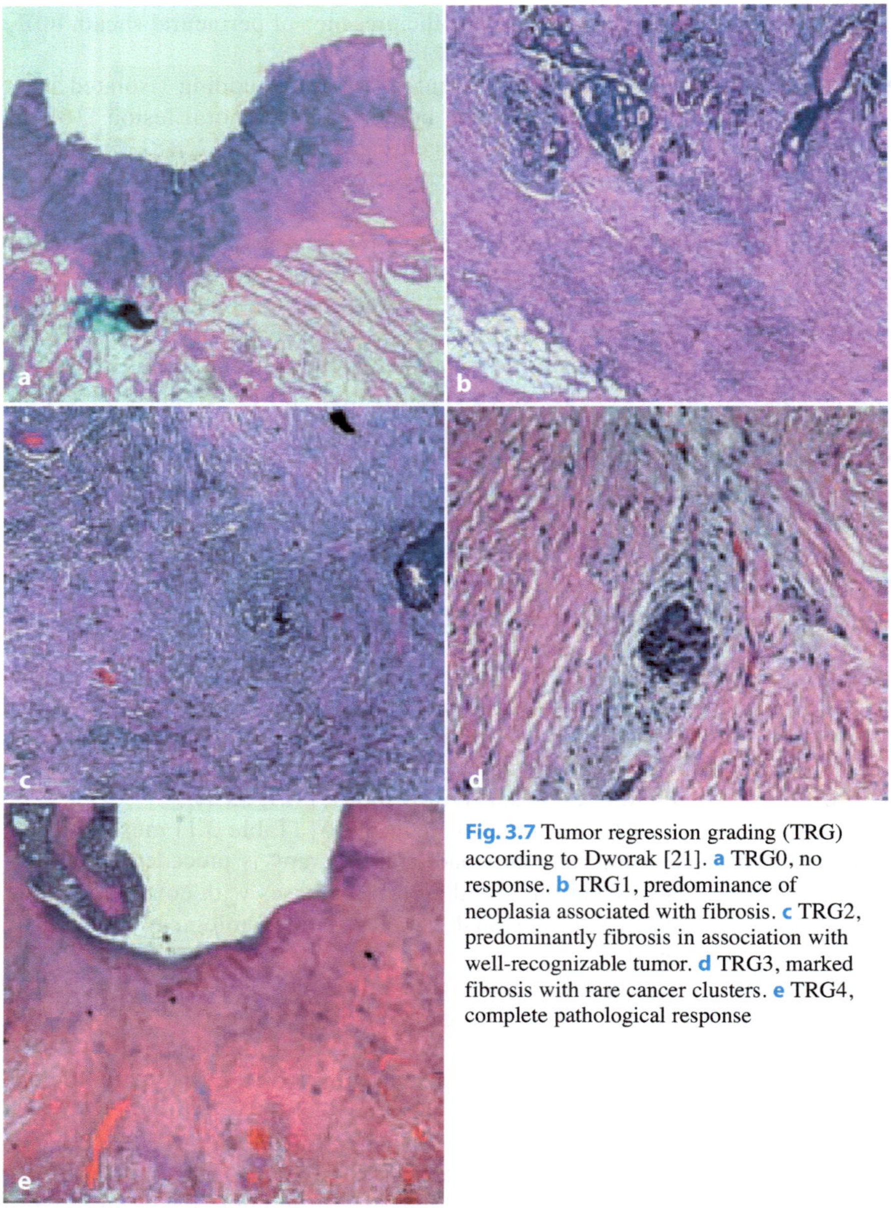

Fig. 3.7 Tumor regression grading (TRG) according to Dworak [21]. **a** TRG0, no response. **b** TRG1, predominance of neoplasia associated with fibrosis. **c** TRG2, predominantly fibrosis in association with well-recognizable tumor. **d** TRG3, marked fibrosis with rare cancer clusters. **e** TRG4, complete pathological response

ing the classification used, because there is no consensus on the positivity cut-off level of the margin (e.g. according to RCP and ADASP [25]: 2 mm, according to AIOM and CAP [5]: 1 mm). It has been suggested that the minimum distance in millimetres of the lesion from the non-peritonealized resection margin should be inserted to avoid any doubt, especially if this distance is between 1 and 2 mm.

In one of our retrospective studies within an audit project at the University Hospital of Trieste in the period 2005-2008, CRM negativity (according to RCP criteria) was observed in 93.5% of patients undergoing TME surgery at the General Surgery Unit of the hospital (de Manzini et al., unpublished data).

For large sessile polyps treated with transanal microsurgery, in which a submucosal invasion is discovered, we suggest using the Kikuchi classification [26], which is useful in risk stratification of lymph node metastases [27] and the subsequent choice of therapy [28]. It is also common practice for this additional information to be given for endoscopic polypectomies, but in our opinion Kikuchi's classification should be used only when the muscolaris propria is present on the sample and in correspondence with the lesion. This is the reference point for a correct evaluation of the extent of the neoplasm in the submucosa (Table 3.2).

The quality of the pathological report depends on several factors:

1. Pre-analytical activity, starting from the information provided by the surgeon, who should never omit fundamental clinical information (first of all any neoadjuvant treatment given) and accuracy in landmarking surgical specimens;
2. Correct handling of the surgical specimen by the pathologist in the sampling phase, which must be aimed at assessing the maximum level of infiltration of the neoplasia, the circumferential resection margin status and the detailed research of all the lymph nodes to provide the most precise pN status;
3. Strict adherence to the guidelines in writing the histopathological report, which must contain not only all the histoprognostic factors useful for stratifying the risk of recurrence of the disease and/or death, but also a concise epicrisis, including histotype, stage (and the extent of postneoadjuvant therapy tumor regression), grading, and margin status. For cases in which metastasis is already present at the moment of the operation, or for those with a high metastatic risk, it is necessary to be able to assess the main molecular markers predicting a response to the targeted molecular therapies. KRAS mutations in exons 12 and 13 are currently the most useful ones. In this case the pathologist is required to take particular care in selecting the area of the neoplasia which is most suitable for molecular investigations, either because of an abundance of well-preserved tumor cells or due to specific morphological characteristics in the case of tumors displaying heterogeneous features.

If there is multidisciplinary collaboration among the various experts with a constant daily exchange of ideas, and also through the instrument of internal auditing, the quality of the treatment can be monitored satisfactorily. This means that any problems that arise during the different steps in the diagnosis and therapy of individual patients can be promptly identified and corrected.

Table 3.1 TNM Rectal staging according to the AJCC Classification, 7th edn. [5]

Primary tumor (T)	
TX	Primary tumor cannot be evaluated
T0	No evidence of primary tumor
Tis	Carcinoma in situ: intraepithelial carcinoma or lamina propria invasion not beyond muscularis mucosae
T1	Tumor invades submucosa
T2	Tumor invades muscularis propria
T3	Tumor invades through the muscularis propria into pericolorectal tissue
T4	Tumor invades other adjacent organs or structures and/or perforates visceral peritoneum
T4a	Tumor penetrates to the surface of visceral peritoneum
T4b	Tumor directly invades or is adherent to other adjacent organs or structures
Regional Lymph Node (N)	
NX	Regional lymph nodes cannot be assessed
N0	No regional lymph nodes metastasis
N1	Metastasis in 1 to 3 regional lymph nodes
N1a	Metastasis in 1 regional lymph nodes
N1b	Metastasis in 2-3 regional lymph nodes
N1c	Tumor deposits (so-called satellites[1]) in the subserosa, or in non peritonealized pericolic/perirectal soft tissue without metastases to regional lymph nodes
N2	Metastasis in 4 or more regional lymph nodes
N2a	Metastasis in 4-6 regional lymph nodes
N2b	Metastasis in 7 o more regional lymph nodes
Distant Metastasis (M)	
M0	No evidence of distant metastasis (no pathological M0; use clinical M to complete stage group)
M1	Distant metastasis
M1a	Metastasis confined to one organ or site (e.g., liver, lung, ovary, non-regional node)
M1b	Metastasis in more than one organ/site or peritoneum (carcinosis)

[1]*Tumor deposits (satellites) in nests or nodules, macroscopic or microscopic, in pericolorectal adipose tissue (lymph drainage area of a primary carcinoma), without evidence of residual lymph node in the nodule, may be an expression of venous invasion (V1/2).*

Table 3.2 Kikuchi classification of submucosal invasion [26]

Sm1	Superior third of the mucosa
Sm1a	Submucosal invasion under ¼ of the tumoral width
Sm1b	Submucosal invasion between ¼ and ½ of the tumoral width
Sm1c	Horizontal affection of the superior third of the submucosa over ½ of the tumoral width
Sm2	Medium third of the submucosa
Sm3	Inferior third of the submucosa

References

1. Quirke P et al (2009) Effect of the plane of surgery achieved on local recurrence in patients with operable rectal cancer: a prospective study using data from the MRC CR07 and NCIC-CTG CO16 randomized clinical trial. Lancet 373:821-828
2. Valentini V et al (2009) Multidisciplinary Rectal Cancer Management: 2nd European Rectal Cancer Consensus Conference (EURECA-CC2). Radiotherapy and Oncology 92:148-63
3. http://www.rcpath.org/index.asp?pageID=1153
4. Quaia E et al (2011) Spectral presaturation inversion recovery MR imaging sequence after gadolinium injection to differentiate fibrotic scar tissue and neoplastic strands in the mesorectal fat in patients undergoing restaging of rectal carcinoma after neoadjuvant chemo- and radiation therapy. Acad Radiol 18:1365-1375
5. Edge SB, Byrd DR, Compton CC (Eds) (2010) AJCC Cancer Staging Manual, 7th edn, Springer, New York, NY
6. Parson HM et al (2011) Association between lymph node evaluation for colon cancer and node positivity over the past 20 years. JAMA 306:1089-1097
7. Funada T et al (2011) Prognostic significance of a new system for categorization of the number of lymph node metastases in gastric cancer.Hepatogastroenterology 58:642-646
8. Petrelli F et al (2011) The emerging issue of ratio of metastatic to resected lymph nodes in gastrointestinal cancers: an overview of literature. Eur J SurgOncol 37:836-847
9. Thomas M et al (2012) Dukes C colorectal cancer: is the metastatic lymph node ratio important? Int J Colorectal Dis 27:309-317
10. Hernanz F et al (2010) The assessment of lymph nodes missed in mesenteric tissue after standard dissection of colorectal cancer specimens. Colorectal Dis 12:e57-e60
11. Caporale A et al (2010) Quantitative investigation of desmoplasia as a prognostic indicator in colorectal cancer. J Invest Surg. Apr 23:105-109
12. Coulson-Thomas VJ et al (2011) Colorectal cancer desmoplastic reaction up-regulates collagen synthesis and restricts cancer cell invasion. Cell Tissue Res 346:223-236
13. Betge J et al (2011) Perineural invasion is a strong and independent predictor of lymph node involvement in colorectal cancer. Dis Colon Rectum 54:e273
14. Peng J et al (2011) Perineural invasion in pT3N0 rectal cancer: the incidence and its prognostic effect. Cancer 117:1415-1421
15. Ceyhan GO et al (2010) The severity of neural invasion is a crucial prognostic factor in rectal cancer independent of neoadjuvant radiochemotherapy. Ann Surg 252:797-804
16. Ueno H et al (2004) Risk factors for an adverse outcome in early invasive colorectal carcinoma. Gastroenterology 127:385-394
17. Ueno H et al (2010) Proposed objective criteria for "grade 3" in early invasive colorectal cancer. Am J Clin Pathol 134:312-22
18. Kajiwara Y et al (2010) Risk factors of nodal involvement in T2 colorectal cancer. Dis Colon Rectum 53:1393-1399
19. Shin JS et al (2011) Histopathological regression grading versus staging of rectal cancer following radiotherapy. Pathology 43:24-30
20. Mandard AM et al (1994) Pathologic assessment of tumor regression after preoperative chemoradiotherapy of esophageal carcinoma. Clinicopathologic correlations. Cancer 73:2680-2686
21. Dworak O et al (1997) Pathological features of rectal cancer after preoperative radiochemotherapy. Int J Colorectal Dis 12:19-23
22. Zaniboni A et al (2004) Adjuvant therapy for stage II colon cancer: an elephant in the living room? Annals of Oncology 15:1310-1318
23. Merkel S et al (2001) High-risk groups of patients with Stage II colon carcinoma. Cancer 92:1435-1443
24. Glimelius B et al (2011) Mesorectal fascia instead of circumferential resection margin in preoperative staging of rectal cancer. J Clin Oncol 29:2142-2143

25. Nagtegaal ID et al (2002) Circumferential margin involvement is still an important predictor of local recurrence in rectal carcinoma: not one millimeter but two millimeters is the limit. Am J Surg Pathol 26:350-357
26. Kikuchi R et al (1995) Management of early invasive colorectal cancer. Risk of recurrence and clinical guidelines. Dis Colon Rectum 38:1286-1295
27. Repici A et al (2009) Endoscopic mucosal resection for early colorectal neoplasia: pathologic basis, procedures and outcome. Dis Colon Rectum 52:1502-1515
28. Ruiz-Tovar J et al (2010) Endoscopic resection as unique treatment for early colorectal cancer. Rev Esp Enferm Dig 102:435-441

Molecular Parameters for Prognostic and Predictive Assessment in Colorectal Cancer

4

Alessandro Carrer, Massimo Giacca and Mauro Giacca

4.1 Introduction

Over the last several years, a large amount of information has been obtained on the molecular and genetic characteristics of colorectal cancer, especially related to the mechanisms of cancer development, invasion, metastasis and response to therapy. Part of this information can be translated into useful molecular testing, which might assist the clinician in classifying patients more effectively and developing personalized therapies. Here we review the molecular characteristics of colorectal cancer, with the specific purpose of highlighting those features currently known to possess prognostic or predictive value.

Colorectal cancer (CRC) is the third most commonly diagnosed type of cancer worldwide and continues to be one of the most fatal [1]. The pace of genetic and molecular discovery in the field of CRC development, progression and metastasis has been impressively rapid over the last few years. Seminal discoveries in the field of hereditary CRC genetics, and later the analysis of global gene expression by microarrays or deep sequencing technologies have generated an impressive amount of information. In turn, this has inevitably raised high expectations that the knowledge gained might permit the identification of molecular markers able to assist the clinician and the surgeon in optimizing and tailoring treatment. This has not necessarily occurred in most cases, and several of the published findings still appear contradictory or redundant. The purpose of this chapter is to summarize the current knowledge on CRC, with

M. Giacca (✉)
Molecular Medicine Laboratory, International Centre for Genetic Engineering and Biotechnology (ICGEB), Trieste, Italy and Department of Medical, Surgical and Health Sciences, University of Trieste,
Trieste, Italy
e-mail: giacca@icgeb.org

N. de Manzini (ed.), *Rectal Cancer*,
Updates in Surgery
DOI: 10.1007/978-88-470-2670-4_4,

the specific purpose of highlighting the molecular information that has actually turned out to be important for prognostic and predictive purposes.

4.2 Molecular Genetics of Colorectal Cancer

Colorectal carcinogenesis represents a paradigm for cancer development due to the successive accumulation of mutations in genes that control epithelial cell growth, differentiation and cell proliferation [2, 3]. Starting from the original hypothesis of multistep carcinogenesis (the so called adenoma-carcinoma sequence [4], involving the subsequent mutations of only a few genes [5]), the most recent determination of cancer genomes has revealed that at least 15 cancer-associated genes may play a role in transformation, and that no less than 80 somatic mutations in exons characterize the genetic landscape of the transformed cells [6, 7]. Some of the detected mutations are inherited and underlie a genetic predisposition to cancer development; most others arise as a constellation of genetic defects in somatic cells and are also present in sporadic CRCs.

It is currently estimated that 15-30% of CRCs have a major hereditary component; of these cases, approximately one-quarter (<5% of all CRC cases) have a Mendelian inheritance due to mutations in single genes [4]. Identification of the mutated alleles in these hereditary tumors have immensely increased our understanding of the genetic defects which also underlie sporadic cancers. The majority of the hereditary cases are attributable to hereditary nonpolyposis colorectal cancer (HNPCC) and the familial adenomatous polyposis (FAP) syndromes.

The genes mutated in HNPCC (Lynch syndrome, which accounts for ~2-5% of all CRCs), are part of a series of genes involved in DNA mismatch repair (MMR), which include MSH2 and MLH1 (70% of cases) and, less frequently, PMS1, PMS2 and GTBP/MSH6 [8]. MMR is a highly conserved - from bacteria to man - strand-specific form of DNA repair that recognizes and repairs base mismatches due to misincorporation, insertion or deletion of nucleotides occurring during DNA replication and recombination or ensuing upon DNA damage [9]. Mutations of the MMR genes account for a peculiar mutator phenotype, which is revealed by marked length variations in microsatellite DNA (microsatellite instability, MSI). HNPCC patients, having inherited a defective MMR gene allele, have a much higher probability of undergoing mutation of the other allele in somatic cells, and manifest the MSI phenotype. As a consequence, the adenoma-carcinoma transition may take 3-5 years in an HNPCC patient, compared to 20-40 years estimated for most sporadic CRCs [4].

A high frequency MSI (MSI-H) phenotype also characterizes approximately 15% of apparently sporadic CRCs [10, 11]. Rather than being due to de novo germline mutations or somatic mutations in MMR genes, this appears to be consequent to the loss of MLH1 gene expression via promoter DNA hypermethylation [8, 12].

On the other hand, FAP accounts for less than 1% of familial CRCs. It is an autosomal dominant syndrome characterized by hundreds to thousands of adenomas that develop in the colon and rectum, with a lifetime probability of malignant transformation approaching 100% [13]. The disease is caused by germline mutations in the adenomatous polyposis coli (APC) gene, a tumor suppressor gene that becomes inactivated by frame-shift or nonsense mutations. APC encodes a ~300 kDa protein involved in the regulation of the Wnt/β-catenin pathway. In particular, APC takes part, together with other cellular proteins such as GSK3β, Axin and CK1α, in the formation of a so-called "destruction complex", which induces proteasomal degradation of β-catenin. Upon Wnt stimulation, this complex is inhibited, and free β-catenin enters the nucleus and activates transcription of several genes, including those coding for factors involved in cell-cell adhesion, cell migration, chromosomal segregation and apoptosis [14]. Thus, the bi-allelic mutation of APC mimics constitutive Wnt signaling in the colon crypt cells.

Deregulation of the Wnt/β-catenin pathway is also a major determinant of sporadic CRC development. Somatic mutation of both APC alleles is an early step in the development of most adenomas; truncations of the gene are detectable in 70-80% of adenomas and carcinomas.

Over the last several years, analysis of sporadic cases of CRC, in addition to the above-described mutations that were originally identified in hereditary CRC, has also highlighted the existence of common mutations in a vast series of other cellular genes. Like many human cancers, three members of the Ras family of the small-G proteins (KRAS, HRAS and NRAS), which are involved in signal transduction from different growth factor receptors (in particular, the epidermal growth factor receptor, EGFR), are mutated in approximately 40% of CRCs [7]. Other common alterations are mutations of the PIK3CA catalytic subunit of the class I PI3Ks (15-25% of cases) and of BRAF, a protein kinase directly activated by RAS, which in turn activates the MAPKs MEK1 and MEK2 (5-10% of CRCs) (Fig. 4.1).

Inactivating mutations and loss of herozygosity (LOH) in tumor suppressor genes are also very frequent. The most common involve the PTEN phosphatase (which is also mutated in the germline of Cowden patients; 10% of CRCs), various members of the TGF-β signaling pathway, including the TGF type II receptor and the SMAD2 and SMAD4 genes, and the FBXW7 gene, which encodes an F-box protein that normally drives degradation of Cyclin E, a cofactor for the CDK2 kinase, which is essential for the transition from the G1 to the S phase of the cell cycle. Finally, approximately 70% of CRCs show LOH for the region of chromosome 17 that encodes the p53 protein, while, in most of these cases, the other allele of the gene is affected by somatic point mutations [3, 4, 8].

A characteristic common to approximately 85% of CRCs is the presence of chromosomal abnormalities, frequently associated with LOH for specific genomic regions. This characteristic chromosome instability (CIN) appears to be a distinctive trait of cancers that do not show MSI-H. The cellular and molecu-

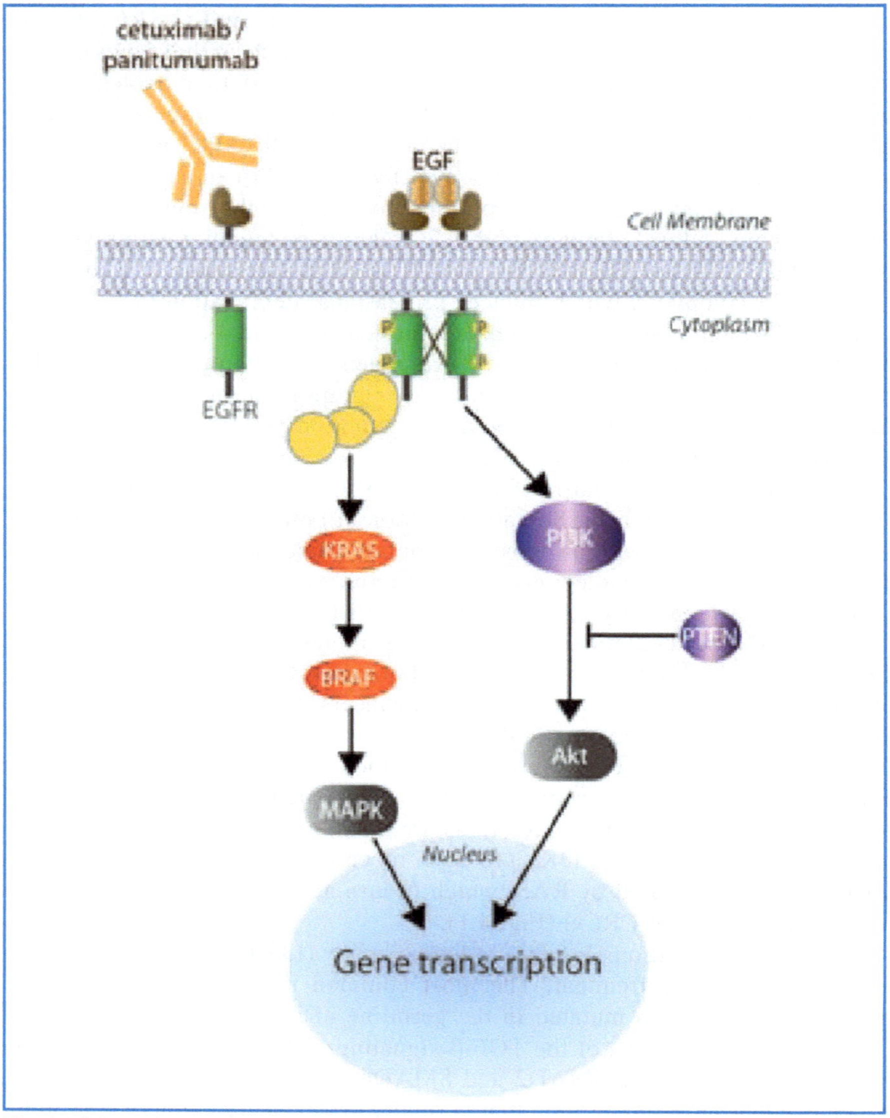

Fig. 4.1 Schematic representation of the EGFR pathway

lar events that determine CIN are still elusive, and are possibly the sum of multiple independent changes, possibly arising as a consequence of the biallelic loss of the APC tumor-suppressor gene, which eventually results in mutations of genes that control mitotic spindle formation or karyokinesis [15, 16]. A surrogate marker of CIN appears to be the partial aneuploidy of the long arm of chromosome 18 (18qLOH), observed in approximately 70% of CRCs and 50% of large, late-stage adenomas. This chromosomal region, among several other genes, encodes for the SMAD2, SMAD4 and SMAD7 factors operating in the TGF-β pathway and for the DCC (Deleted in Colorectal Carcinoma) gene [4].

Finally, approximately 15% of CRCs show a characteristic epigenetic abnormality consisting in hypermethylation of CpG islands at gene promoters. In mammalian genomes, more than 80% of cytosines at the CpG dinucleotide are modified by methylation, with the exception of highly CpG-dense islands, mainly located in the promoters of approximately 50% of the genes. In CRC cells, there is a generalized decrease in the total level of methylation of the genome, in any case accompanied by the selective methylation of several CpG islands and the consequent epigenetic silencing of the neighboring genes [17]. Modification of the normal DNA methylation pattern defines the so-called CpG island hypermethylation phenotype (CIMP), which ultimately modifies the expression of various genes essential for cell differentiation and cell-fate determination [18]. The CIMP phenotype contributes to the global deregulation of the gene expression profile that is commonly observed by analyzing the CRC transcriptome.

4.3 Molecular Markers for Early Cancer Detection

While colonscopy is the most accurate procedure for CRC screening, it is expensive, has poor patient compliance and can be associated with procedure-related complications. In contrast, fecal occult blood testing (FOBT) is inexpensive but has low sensitivity and specificity. Instead, detection of the specific genomic changes due to DNA hypermethylation could be used for specific, sensitive and noninvasive testing for early cancer detection, especially because CIMP already shows development in early polyp lesions. Assays start from genomic DNA extracted from stool or plasma samples and detect the presence of methylated CpGs upon quantitative PCR amplification of the promoter regions of specific genes. Among the genes considered so far are those coding for Vimentin, Septin, AKAP12, TFPI2 or SPG20 [17, 19]. Of these, stool-based methylated Vimentin detection is now an early detection, clinically validated test for colorectal cancer, commercially available in the U.S (ColoSure™) [20]. This assay is reported to have a sensitivity of 83% and a specificity of 82%, with approximately equal sensitivity in patients with stage I to III colorectal cancer [21].

4.4 Molecular Markers for Prognostic Assessment

A vast number of studies have addressed the possibility of exploiting the existence of common genetic and molecular features in CRC patients (presence of MSI, CIN, CIMP, LOH at defined loci and existence of specific DNA mutations) for prognostic purposes. The overall outcome of these studies is schematically summarized in Table 4.I.

Table 4.1 Synoptic view of the most frequent molecular and genetic alterations found in CRC and their use as prognostic or predictive markers

Molecular characteristics	Prognostic value	Predictive value
Genetic and epigenetic alterations		
Mutation of MMR genes (MSI-H phenotype)	Favorable - strong evidence	Unfavorable for 5-FU; uncertain for irinotecan
CIN	Unfavorable - strong evidence	
18qLOH (positive correlation with CIN and negative with MSI)	Unfavorable - moderate evidence	Possibly unfavorable
CIMP (correlates with presence of BRAF and KRAS mutations)	Unfavorable - value as an independent marker uncertain	
Mutations of specific genes		
Mutation of APC		
Mutation of KRAS	Unfavorable in advanced disease - clinical use uncertain	Strong predictor of inefficacy of anti-EGFR therapies
Mutation of PI3CA	Unfavorable - clinical use uncertain	
Mutation of BRAF	Unfavorable - clinical use uncertain	Mutation V600E predicts resistance to anti-EGFR therapies
Mutation of PTEN		Mutation predicts resistance to anti-EGFR therapies
Amplification of EGFR, CDK8 or c-MYC		Clinical value uncertain
17qLOH and/or p53 mutation		Variant Pro72 sensitizes cells to 5-FU; clinical value uncertain
Levels of gene expression		
Oncotype DX Colon Cancer Test (7 genes) and ColoPrint (8 genes)	Predict risk of recurrence	Clinical value uncertain
miRNA expression pattern	Research stage only Prognostic significance uncertain	
TFAP2ε		Low expression predictive of unresponsiveness to 5-FU
EGFR		Overexpression predictive of unresponsiveness to cetuximab
VEGF-A, LDH5		Overexpression predictive of poor response to bevacizumab and vatalanib

(*cont.*) ↓

Genetic polymorphisms		
DPD, MTHFR		Polymorphisms predict sensitivity to 5-FU
GST-P1		Polymorphisms predict sensitivity to oxaliplatin
UGT1A1		Presence of UGT1A1*28 associated with drug-induced neutropenia
Thymidylate synthase (TS)		Polymorphisms in the non-coding regions associated with decreased response to 5-FU
ERCC-1		Polymorphisms predict sensitivity to oxaliplatin
VEGF-A		Polymorphisms in the promoter region affect levels of expression and response to bevacizumab
Infiltration by circulating cells		
CTLs (extent of CTL infiltration correlates with MSI status)	CTL infiltration favorable - negatively correlated with lymph node metastasis	
T-regs	Presence of T-regs unfavorable	
Myeloid cells		Extent of tumor infiltration negative correlates with efficacy of anti-angiogenic therapy
Other characteristics		
Intratumoral hypoxia		Predicts resistance to 5-FU and oxaliplatin
Immature and aberrant tumor vasculature		Predicts resistance to chemotherapy - Difficult to assess in vivo

4.4.1 Prognostic Value of Genetic and Epigenetic Tumor Characteristics

The most common, mutually exclusive, specific genetic features at the basis of colon carcinogenesis are MSI and CIN. MSI has a frequency of 15% and is defined by the presence of at least 30% unstable loci in a panel of 5-10 loci consisting of mono- and dinucleotide tracts [22]. CIN on the other hand is found in as many as 85% CRCs and is defined as the presence of numerical chromosome changes and structural aberrations; it is typically assessed by flow cytometry [23].

These two characteristics readily distinguish normal from transformed colonic epithelium and are discriminant in the prognosis of CRC, since several clinical studies and their meta-analyses have extensively documented that CIN-positive tumors carry a worse prognosis than MSI-positive ones [24, 25]. The hazard ratio for overall survival was estimated to be 0.65 for MSI CRCs vs. 1.45 for CIN CRC [23]. Despite the association of MSI and CIN with prognosis, however, these determinations have not yet entered routine testing for clinical decision making [26, 27].

Another prognostic marker is the deletion of the long arm of chromosome 18 (18qLOH). CRC patients with 18qLOH have a worse prognosis compared with patients with tumors without 18qLOH [26, 27]. There is a strict correlation of 18qLOH with CIN and an inverse correlation with MSI. As a consequence, it is still unclear whether 18qLOH is a truly independent maker for prognostic assessment or rather a surrogate marker for CIN/MSI assessment [23].

A third epigenetic instability marker, after CIN and MSI, is CIMP, commonly defined as the CpG methylation of at least three loci from a selected panel of five CpG islands [23]. Retrospective studies have indicated that CIMP is a negative marker for CRC progression and survival; however, its prognostic value as an independent marker is uncertain at the moment, especially because patients with CIMP also carry BRAF or KRAS mutations [26].

4.4.2 Prognostic Value of Individual Genetic Mutations

Among the specific genetic mutations detected in CRC patients, those of the genes coding for proteins involved in signal transduction from the receptor tyrosine kinases and the EGFR in particular, have been extensively investigated. These include mutations in KRAS, BRAF and PIK3CA [28-30] (Fig. 4.1). There is now limited evidence that the presence of mutations in KRAS codons 12 and 13 (which are validated predictive markers for treatment with EGFR inhibitors; cf. below), PIK3CA and BRAF are prognostically unfavorable, especially in advanced diseases; however, the clinical usefulness of these findings is uncertain at the moment [23].

4.4.3 Prognostic Value of Gene Expression Profiling

Over the last few years, a vast series of studies have assessed global expression profiles of CRCs by microarrays or, more modernly, by deep RNA sequencing, or have analyzed the levels of expression of various subsets of individual genes, with the ultimate purpose of establishing possible correlations between gene expression and prognosis.

In particular, two gene expression profiling diagnostic tests have been the object of important clinical studies. Both tests determine the risk of recurrence and relapse-free survival of colorectal cancers in stage II and III after surgical resection. This area of interest appears to be of particular importance, since better risk stratification is needed in a phase of disease when the risk of recurrence exists and the indications for chemotherapy are controversial. The Oncotype DX® Colon Cancer Test has been commercially available since January 2010, while the ColoPrint® assay was clinically and technically validated in 2012.

The Oncotype DX® Colon Cancer Test, similar to the by now clinically validated Oncotype DX® Breast Cancer Assay, uses fixed, paraffin-embedded primary tumor tissues and analyses, using RT-PCR, seven cancer-related genes selected from a panel of 761 genes recurring in CRCs. Of these seven genes, three are involved in cell proliferation (MK167, MYBL2 and MYC), three are associated with activated stroma (BGN, INHBA and FAP), and one is part of the DNA damage response (GADD45B). Expression values for these seven genes are normalized according to the levels of five reference genes, and the values are then elaborated to provide an individualized recurrence risk score [31, 32]. The ColoPrint® test, devised to follow the validated breast cancer test MammaPrint®, is a microarray assay which analyses the levels of expression of 18 unique genes associated with prognostic significance for tumor recurrence in patients who have undergone surgical resection for stage II or III colorectal cancer. Patients are divided into high and low risk of recurrence. ColoPrint® facilitates the identification of patients with stage II disease who may be safely managed without use of chemotherapy [32, 33].

As far as the expression of specific subsets of genes is concerned, different studies have aimed at identifying markers that could predict the metastatic potential, especially since deaths caused by CRC can mostly be attributed to visceral metastasis. One study identified PCSK7, which codes for the proprotein convertase subtilisin/kexin type 7, as the top upregulated gene in metastatic tumors [34]. In contrast, the expression of several genes appears to be deregulated in node involvement, including tumor suppressor genes (ST7, BAP1), OAS1 and NTRK2, PRSS8 (encoding for the prostasin serine protease) and PSMA, which was also related to node metastasis in prostate cancer [34, 35]. The expression of FOXC2, instead, was reported to be directly proportional to the aggressiveness of node metastasis in CRCs [36]. Finally, one study also analyzed the levels of expression of approximately 30 genes involved in angiogenesis and lymphangiogenesis, and identified the levels of Plexin-A1 and stromal cell-derived factor 1 (SDF-1) as predictors to discriminate between tumor and paired normal mucosa, the former being overexpressed and the latter downregulated in tumors [37]. Collectively, these studies have provided important insights into the mechanisms of tumor development and metastatic spread. For example, it is now clear that gene expression in primitive tumors, visceral metastasis and lymph node metastasis is largely dissimilar, indicating that the two metastatic processes are biologically different and that the metastatic cells are affected by the microenvironment where they become established [38]. However, the very high inter-patient, intra-study and inter-study variability prevents the use of individual gene expression for prognostic purposes at the moment.

An essential level of gene regulation, the importance of which has been increasingly appreciated over the last few years, is the control of mRNA levels by the cellular microRNA (miRNA) network. MiRNAs as small (20-22 nt long), noncoding RNAs, produced by processing the primary transcripts of over 1,000 cellular genes. The miRNA network impacts on all aspects of mammalian biology, including cancer development and spread [39]. MiRNAs may also represent a novel class of prognostic and possible predictive biomarkers, especially because a few of them are released, and can be detected, in blood and feces [40, 41]. Although several miRNAs have been reported to be differentially expressed in specimens from CRC patients, very limited validation is currently available. As a consequence, it is too early to draw conclusions as to the extent to which some miRNAs might actually translate into specific biomarkers useful in clinical practice.

4.4.4 Prognostic Value of Immune Cell Infiltration

Human solid cancers are invariably infiltrated by various lymphoid cell populations. A direct relationship between the intratumoral presence of cytotoxic T lymphocytes (CTLs) and CRC patient survival has been detected in several analyses; interestingly, CTL infiltration appears to be more marked in MSI-H tumors [42] and is inversely proportional to lymph node metastasis [26].

Another lymphoid cell population that has been widely investigated in recent years are the CD4+ CD25+ T-regulatory (T-reg) cells. The presence of infiltrating Forkhead Box P3-Positive (FOXP3) T-regs has been associated with a worse prognosis in CRC patients, probably due to their function in suppressing antitumor immunity. Different studies have indicate that T-regs are markers of shorter patient survival and predictors of recurrence when associated with decreased levels of CD8+ CTLs [43-45].

4.5 Molecular Markers Predicting Response to Therapy

Adjuvant and neoadjuvant chemotherapy using 5-FluoroUracil (5-FU)-based regimens is often indicated for patients with stage II or stage III disease (www.asco.gov; www.cancer.gov). Clinical and biochemical parameters, such as perforation, obstruction, local and lymph node invasion, or circulating levels of carcinoembryonic antigen (CEA) have clear prognostic value, but they do not predict which patients are likely to benefit from chemotherapy [10]. In particular, approximately 25 to 30% of newly diagnosed CRC cases have node-negative (stage II) disease; with surgery alone, the overall survival at 5 years of these patients is about 80% [46]. Adjuvant chemotherapy offers most of these phase II patients a minimal incremental benefit, with improvement in survival being less than 5% [32]. Thus, defining the genetic or molecular characteristics of the subset of patients with high-risk stage II disease who benefit from adjuvant regimens appears particularly important. The most important results of the studies so far conducted are summarized in Table 4.1 and reported below.

4.5.1 Predictive Value of Genetic and Epigenetic Tumor Characteristics

Both prospective [47-49] and retrospective [50, 51] studies performed in stage II CRC patients have suggested that MSI-H is a negative predictor of 5-FU response. Furthermore, there is also evidence that 5-FU-based therapies might even be detrimental for some MSI-H stage II individuals [47]. Therefore, although neither ASCO nor the European Group on Tumor Markers currently recommends MSI testing to guide treatment selection, it might reasonably be expected that such a recommendation will be included in the guidelines in the near future. Fortunately, however, the presence of MSI-H itself has a good prognostic value for stage II patients, such as not to justify the administration of adjuvant chemotherapy. In terms of the specific response to Irinotecan, on the other hand, there is still controversy on the role of MSI-H determination [52-54].

As far as 18qLOH is concerned, this marker appears to be a powerful predictor of patients with adverse response to 5-FU-based therapy [55]. The observation that reduced levels of SMAD4, a gene located within the 18q region, are associated with a worse response to 5-FU is consistent with this conclusion [56].

4.5.2 Predictive Value of Specific Genetic Variations

As already discussed above, the EGFR pathway is often constitutively activated in advanced CRC, often correlating with more aggressive tumor phenotypes, and is thus a well-conceived target for anti-cancer therapies. To date, two monoclonal antibodies (cetuximab – Erbitux®– and panitumumab – Vectibix®–) have been approved for use in combinatorial regimens (Fig. 4.1) [57, 58]. Their effectiveness, however, seems clear in only a small subset of stage IV CRC patients [59]. Some evidence has suggested that EGFR gene copy number might correlate with improved response to both monoclonal antibodies [60], but major technical issues hamper the clinical application of this determination.

In patients resistant to cetuximab and panitumumab, point mutations in EGFR are uncommon, unlike the situation with other types of cancers. In contrast, mutations in KRAS account for approximately 50-60% of these resistances [26]. Genetic testing for KRAS is now currently required by both the FDA and the European Medicines Agency (EMEA) to select CRC patients who would benefit from anti-EGFR therapies, and clearly stands as one the brightest examples of the potential usefulness of a biomarker to predict drug responsiveness [61]. In spite of the clear predictive value of KRAS mutations, however, no more than 50% of wild-type KRAS patients objectively respond to anti-EGFR therapies, possibly as a consequence of alterations in other members of the EGFR pathway [61].

Like KRAS, BRAF is a protein kinase frequently mutated in many cancer types. The vast majority of BRAF mutations occur at a single hotspot at position 1799, resulting in a Valine to Glutamic acid substitution (commonly referred to as V600E) [62]; as a consequence, the BRAF mutation is an ideal biomarker for routine clinical use. Both retrospective and prospective studies have in fact confirmed an association between V600E and poor response to anti-EGFR therapies [63-65]. BRAF genotyping has recently been included in the major guidelines for the selection of patients scheduled to undergo anti-EGFR therapies.

Preclinical evidence suggests that PTEN deficiency also determines resistance to anti-EGFR drugs [66, 67]. Analysis of PTEN status by tissue immunohistochemistry has indeed indicated that almost half of CRCs have impaired PTEN expression [68, 69]. Interestingly, however, only PTEN status at the level of metastasis appeared to correlate with efficacy of cetuximab treatment.

Finally, although not unequivocally, there is evidence that response to 5-FU is associated to retention of wild-type p53 status, at least for stage III patients [70]. In the p53 protein, a common polymorphism at codon 72 distinguishes two protein variants (Arg72 or Pro72), which have different biochemical properties [71]. The presence of the Pro72 variant might contribute to sensitize tumor cells to 5-FU [72]. Despite decades of work assessing the predominant role of p53 in tumor biology, however, the establishment of this protein as a biomarker is seriously hampered by major technical issues that can be overcome only with systematic gene sequencing, an approach still far from clinical routine.

4.5.3 Predictive Value of Gene Expression Profiling

Over the last few years, several small studies have profiled gene expression in CRC surgical specimens to identify possible gene combinations that might have prognostic or predictive value [37, 73-77]. Overall, these studies have led to inconclusive results, possibly due their relatively small scale, except for the fact that they indicate that there is very wide patient-to-patient variation in the levels of expression of most of the analysed genes, which essentially prevents the identification of potentially universal predictive markers. Unlike the commercially available OncoType DX® Breast Cancer, or the MammaPrint® assays, which provide both prognostic and predictive information for women with breast cancer, the above-described OncoType DX® Colon Cancer and ColoPrint® tests for gene expression profiling in CRC provide prognostic information, but their capacity to predict response to therapy appears highly uncertain at the moment [32].

As far as the analysis of individual genes is concerned, a particularly promising observation was that low expression of SMAD4 (a gene located in the long arm of chromosome 18) was associated with poor responsiveness to 5-FU-based adjuvant chemotherapy [55], especially since this observation was in line with previous data linking drug efficacy to 18qLOH [78]. However, neither low expression of SMAD4 nor 18qLOH has been consistently confirmed in subsequent studies. Enthusiasm for gene expression as a predictive biomarker has very recently been revitalized by a study showing that the low expression of Transcription Factor AP-2 epsilon (TFAP2ε), possibly consequent to promoter hypermethylation, was predictive of unresponsiveness to 5-FU [79].

Interestingly, analysis of gene expression appears rather to have an exploitable value to predict the effectiveness of a series of new generation drugs, essentially EGFR and VEGF inhibitors. As already discussed, responsiveness to anti-EGFR monoclonal antibodies (i.e., cetuximab) is well predicted by mutations in effector genes in the EGF pathway, mainly KRAS and BRAF. As a general rule, mutations that activate these genes curtail the effect of EGFR inhibitors [27]. However, there is a subset of tumors that are not sensitive to EGFR therapies despite the apparent lack of mutations of KRAS or BRAF. A few studies have indicated that, in these cases, resistance might be the consequence of overexpression of EGFR or EGFR ligands [80, 81]. Similarly, high expression of VEGF-A or LDH5 (lactate de-hydrogenase) might account for the poor response to the angiogenesis inhibitors bevacizumab and vatalanib, respectively [82, 83]. The clinical usefulness of these observations remains undefined at the moment.

4.5.4 Genetic Polymorphisms Affecting Drug Efficacy

The vast majority of chemotherapy regimens are designed as 5-FU-based therapies, hence its associated toxicity is a relevant matter in clinical management. Nearly the entire 5-FU content in the organism is catabolized by the enzyme dehydro-pyrimidine dehydrogenase (DPD). Expression of this enzyme varies significantly within the population, with a small fraction (less than 5%) being partially or totally deficient [84]. Since impairment of DPD function can lead to life-threatening 5-FU toxicity [85], it appears important to determine DPD status. Clinical application of this concept, however, is rendered difficult by the fact that about 30 different SNPs have been associated to DPD deficiency.

The role of methylene-tetrahydrofolate reductase (MTHFR) in indirectly increasing sensitivity to 5-FU is on the other hand less clear [27]. In this case, two common polymorphisms that affect MTHFR activity (C677T and A1298C) have been shown to increase responsiveness to 5-FU [86]. Despite the obvious interest in predicting 5-FU toxicity, none of these findings has so far been translated into the clinic.

Oxaliplatin, like other platinum derivatives, undergoes hepatic detoxification, through various enzymes mainly belonging to the glutathione-S-transferase (GST) family. Among these isoenzymes, GST-P1 is the most prominent in oxaliplatin catabolism. Two well-characterized polymorphisms in the coding region of the protein have been shown to significantly decrease GST-P1 activity [87]. These substitutions, which occur in approximately 15% of the entire population, severely impair drug metabolism [88], eventually resulting in oxaliplatin-induced neuropathy. Toxicity, however, appears to have importance only at high drug dosage [89].

The active metabolite of irinotecan, SN-38, is mainly detoxified by UDP-glucuronosyl-transferase-1-A1 (UGT1A1). Several studies have reported an association between a particular polymorphism (UGT1A1*28) and drug-induced neutropenia, due to reduced enzyme activity resulting in insufficient drug clearance [90]. In 2005, the American Food and Drug Administration (FDA) approved a commercial test for UGT1A1, to assist in the correct choice of irinotecan dosage [23]; the practical usefulness of this test, however, is limited by the fact that the irinotecan doses administered in combination regimens (such as standard FOLFIRI) have negligible toxicity.

Besides drug metabolism, another set of genetic polymorphisms affect the levels of expression or the function of the factors targeted by the drugs. The main target of the 5-FU active metabolite (5-FdUMP) is the enzyme thymidylate synthase (TS). A few polymorphisms located in the promoter region or in the 3' untranslated portion of the mRNA are known to modify the levels of expression of the TS gene and have been variously associated to increased or decreased response to 5-FU [91]. Multiple clinical trials are currently ongoing to further define the clinical usefulness of these findings.

Oxaliplatin mainly exerts its activity through the formation of DNA adducts, that eventually impede DNA replication but are tentatively repaired by the cellular DNA repair proteins. Expression of one of these proteins, ERCC-1, was suggested to be predictive of drug response [92, 93], a possibility that is now being explored by an ongoing clinical trial (OPTIMOX2) [94].

Finally, bevacizumab is a monoclonal antibody that specifically targets the Vascular Endothelial Growth Factor (VEGF), approved for the combinatorial treatment of advanced, refractory CRC, in which it has so far shown a modest and rather disappointing performance [49]. A polymorphism in the promoter region of VEGF (C to T change at position -1498) appears to modulate host VEGF levels, with the C/C allelic combination significantly correlating with amelioration of the clinical outcome when bevacizumab is administered along with standard FOLFIRI regimen [95].

Collectively, these findings unveil the importance of SNP determination as an important tool to predict response to therapy. It is still early days, but it can easily be predicted that, like other malignancies, SNP genotyping will become an integral part of the clinical management of CRC patients in the near future.

4.5.5 The Tumor Microenvironment and its Predictive Potential

Formation of an abnormal vasculature and presence of white blood cells are two features that invariably accompany the development of many types of solid cancers. In particular, tumors are invariably infiltrated by a set of monocytic cells of myeloid origin, among them the tumor-associated macrophages, TAMs, which exert a pro-angiogenic function, or the myeloid-derived suppressor cells (MDSCs), which suppress the host immune response [96]. In mouse pre-clinical models, the extent of this myeloid cell infiltration correlates with poor responsiveness to anti-VEGF treatment [97]. In keeping with the poor clinical success of bevacizumab, colorectal tumors are known to abundantly mobilize these cells through the secretion of GM-CSF [98]. Thus, the extent of myeloid cell infiltration, or the circulating levels of GM-CSF, or those of other angiogenic factors that might overcome VEGF inhibition, are currently being assessed as possible markers to guide patient selection for anti-VEGF treatments.

Another common characteristics of solid tumors, particularly including CRC, is the presence of intratumoral hypoxia. Chronic low oxygen tensions activate a variegated molecular program, crucially orchestrated by the hypoxia-inducible factor 1alpha (HIF-1α), which eventually leads to chemoresistance, radioresistance, angiogenesis and invasiveness of malignant cells. The first evidence that hypoxic conditioning desensitizes tumor cells to 5-FU was produced more than two decades ago [99], and there is now ample pre-clinical evidence that hypoxia predicts both 5-FU and oxaliplatin chemoresistance. The actual translation of these findings to the clinic is however more problematic, especially because of significant inconsistencies among the different methodologies used to quantify hypoxia in tissues.

The establishment of a chronic tumor-associated hypoxic state is directly linked to the status of the tumor vasculature, which is characterized by a poor association with perivascular mural cells (smooth muscle cells or pericytes), increased ramification and stagnant blood flow [100]. Such an inefficient and leaky vasculature represents a major obstacle to drug penetration, and its "normalization" therefore is now regarded as an important strategy to increase drug responsiveness. This is of particular relevance in the case of CRC, where bevacizumab has been demonstrated to induce vessel normalization in some settings, possibly expressing its effectiveness only in combinatorial regimens [101]. In this respect, however, the quantitative determination of vessel normalization appears difficult, as all the proposed techniques (MRI, PET, ultrasound, CT, immunostaining) still suffer from significant limitations [101].

4.6 Peculiarity of Rectal Cancer

In clinical practice, locally advanced rectal cancer is commonly considered biologically very similar to CRC, as it has a comparable molecular evolution and often carries overlapping molecular alterations [23]. However, there is no demonstration that the events leading to cancer development are superimposable in every colorectal region. In addition, pathological and molecular evidence demonstrating how colon and rectal cancers carry different characteristics is increasing.

A large randomized trial has recently started to validate the most important CRC molecular markers specifically in rectal cancer (www.clinicaltrials.gov; ID:NCT00835055). So far, the available evidence indicates that both MSI and BRAF mutations are significantly more frequent in colon cancer, but only if we compare the right-sided ones to rectal neoplasms [102-104]. While CIMP+ status can reach 40% in proximal colon tumors, approximately only 10% distal colorectal cancers are CIMP+ [102, 103, 105]. On the other hand, there is controversy concerning the presence of KRAS mutations [102-104]. The frequency of p53 mutations is higher in rectal and left colon cancer (40-60%) than in proximal CRC (25-40%), and has independent prognostic value; the types of mutations, however, appear superimposable [106, 107].

A number of studies have also analyzed the expression profiles of cancers from the distal and proximal parts of the colon, and from the rectum. These studies have reinforced the recognition that colon cancer and rectal cancer can develop through different oncogenic events, especially comparing right-sided CRCs to left-sided and rectal CRCs. Over 60 genes have been found, the expression of which is different between left- and right-sided CRCs [108, 109]. Whether some of the genes specifically expressed in rectal cancer might used as prognostic or predictive markers in the future, is a matter that must await further investigation.

Acknowledgments The authors are grateful to Suzanne Kerbavcic for excellent editorial assistance. This work was supported by Advanced Grant 20090506 from the European Research Council (ERC) to M.G.

References

1. Jemal A, Bray F, Center MM et al (2011) Global cancer statistics. CA Cancer J Clin 61:69-90
2. Michor F, Iwasa Y, Lengauer C et al (2005) Dynamics of colorectal cancer. Semin Cancer Biol 15:484-93
3. Jass JR (2006) Colorectal cancer: a multipathway disease. Crit Rev Oncol 12:273-87
4. Fearon ER (2011) Molecular genetics of colorectal cancer. Annu Rev Pathol 6:479-507
5. Fearon ER, Vogelstein B (1990) A genetic model for colorectal tumorigenesis. Cell 61:759-767
6. Sjoblom T, Jones S, Wood LD et al (2006) The consensus coding sequences of human breast and colorectal cancers. Science 314:268-74
7. Wood LD, Parsons DW, Jones S et al (2007) The genomic landscapes of human breast and colorectal cancers. Science 318:1108-1113
8. Rustgi AK (2007) The genetics of hereditary colon cancer. Genes Dev 21:2525-2538
9. Kunkel TA, Erie DA (2005) DNA mismatch repair. Annu Rev Biochem 74:681-710
10. Gangadhar T, Schilsky RL, Medscape (2010) Molecular markers to individualize adjuvant therapy for colon cancer. Nat Rev Clin Oncol 7:318-325
11. Vilar E, Gruber SB (2010) Microsatellite instability in colorectal cancer-the stable evidence. Nat Rev Clin Oncol 7:153-162
12. Sinicrope FA, Sargent DJ (2012) Molecular Pathways: Microsatellite Instability in Colorectal Cancer: Prognostic, Predictive, and Therapeutic Implications. Clin Cancer Res 18:1506-1512
13. Galiatsatos P, Foulkes WD (2006) Familial adenomatous polyposis. Am J Gastroenterol 101:385-398
14. Brocardo M, Henderson BR (2008) APC shuttling to the membrane, nucleus and beyond. Trends Cell Biol 18:587-596
15. Grady WM (2004) Genomic instability and colon cancer. Cancer Metastasis Rev 23:11-27
16. Barber TD, McManus K, Yuen KW et al (2008) Chromatid cohesion defects may underlie chromosome instability in human colorectal cancers. Proc Natl Acad Sci U S A 105:3443-3448
17. Kim MS, Lee J, Sidransky D (2010) DNA methylation markers in colorectal cancer. Cancer Metastasis Rev 29:181-206
18. Irizarry RA, Ladd-Acosta C, Wen B et al (2009) The human colon cancer methylome shows similar hypo- and hypermethylation at conserved tissue-specific CpG island shores. Nat Genet 41:178-186
19. Lind GE, Raiborg C, Danielsen SA et al (2011) SPG20, a novel biomarker for early detection of colorectal cancer, encodes a regulator of cytokinesis. Oncogene 30:3967-3978
20. Ned RM, Melillo S, Marrone M (2011) Fecal DNA testing for Colorectal Cancer Screening: the ColoSure test. PLoS Curr 3:RRN1220.
21. Itzkowitz S, Brand R, Jandorf L et al (2008) A simplified, noninvasive stool DNA test for colorectal cancer detection. Am J Gastroenterol 103:2862-2870
22. Boland CR, Thibodeau SN, Hamilton SR et al (1998) A National Cancer Institute Workshop on Microsatellite Instability for cancer detection and familial predisposition: development of international criteria for the determination of microsatellite instability in colorectal cancer. Cancer Res 58:5248-5257
23. Pritchard CC, Grady WM (2011) Colorectal cancer molecular biology moves into clinical practice. Gut 60:116-129
24. Walther A, Houlston R, Tomlinson I (2008) Association between chromosomal instability and prognosis in colorectal cancer: a meta-analysis. Gut 57:941-950
25. Popat S, Hubner R, Houlston RS (2005) Systematic review of microsatellite instability and colorectal cancer prognosis. J Clin Oncol 23:609-618
26. Deschoolmeester V, Baay M, Specenier P et al (2010) A review of the most promising biomarkers in colorectal cancer: one step closer to targeted therapy. Oncologist 15:699-731

27. Walther A, Johnstone E, Swanton C et al (2009) Genetic prognostic and predictive markers in colorectal cancer. Nat Rev Cancer 9:489-499
28. Ogino S, Meyerhardt JA, Irahara N et al (2009) KRAS mutation in stage III colon cancer and clinical outcome following intergroup trial CALGB 89803. Clin Cancer Res 15:7322-7329
29. Roth AD, Tejpar S, Delorenzi M et al (2010) Prognostic role of KRAS and BRAF in stage II and III resected colon cancer: results of the translational study on the PETACC-3, EORTC 40993, SAKK 60-00 trial. J Clin Oncol 28:466-474
30. Tol J, Nagtegaal ID, Punt CJ (2009) BRAF mutation in metastatic colorectal cancer. N Engl J Med 361:98-99
31. Clark-Langone KM, Sangli C, Krishnakumar J, Watson D (2010) Translating tumor biology into personalized treatment planning: analytical performance characteristics of the Oncotype DX Colon Cancer Assay. BMC Cancer 10:691
32. Kelley RK, Venook AP (2011) Prognostic and predictive markers in stage II colon cancer: is there a role for gene expression profiling? Clin Colorectal Cancer 10:73-80
33. Salazar R, Roepman P, Capella G et al (2011) Gene expression signature to improve prognosis prediction of stage II and III colorectal cancer. J Clin Oncol 29:17-24
34. Bertucci F, Salas S, Eysteries S et al (2004) Gene expression profiling of colon cancer by DNA microarrays and correlation with histoclinical parameters. Oncogene 23:1377-1391
35. Watanabe T, Kobunai T, Tanaka T et al (2009) Gene expression signature and the prediction of lymph node metastasis in colorectal cancer by DNA microarray. Dis Colon Rectum 52:1941-1948
36. Watanabe T, Kobunai T, Yamamoto Y et al (2011) Gene expression of mesenchyme forkhead 1 (FOXC2) significantly correlates with the degree of lymph node metastasis in colorectal cancer. Int Surg 96:207-216
37. Carrer A, Zacchigna S, Balani A et al (2008) Expression profiling of angiogenic genes for the characterisation of colorectal carcinoma. Eur J Cancer 44:1761-1769
38. Chiang AC, Massague J (2008) Molecular basis of metastasis. N Engl J Med 359:2814-2823
39. Bartel DP (2009) MicroRNAs: target recognition and regulatory functions. Cell 136:215-233
40. Link A, Balaguer F, Shen Y et al (2010) Fecal MicroRNAs as novel biomarkers for colon cancer screening. Cancer Epidemiol Biomarkers Prev 19:1766-1774
41. Pu XX, Huang GL, Guo HQ et al (2010) Circulating miR-221 directly amplified from plasma is a potential diagnostic and prognostic marker of colorectal cancer and is correlated with p53 expression. J Gastroenterol Hepatol 25:1674-1680
42. Atreya I, Schimanski CC, Becker C et al (2007) The T-box transcription factor eomesodermin controls CD8 T cell activity and lymph node metastasis in human colorectal cancer. Gut 56:1572-1578
43. Betts G, Jones E, Junaid S et al (2011) Suppression of tumor-specific CD4+ T cells by regulatory T cells is associated with progression of human colorectal cancer. Gut, in press
44. Frey DM, Droeser RA, Viehl CT et al (2010) High frequency of tumor-infiltrating FOXP3(+) regulatory T cells predicts improved survival in mismatch repair-proficient colorectal cancer patients. Int J Cancer 126:2635-2643
45. Salama P, Phillips M, Grieu F et al (2009) Tumor-infiltrating FOXP3+ T regulatory cells show strong prognostic significance in colorectal cancer. J Clin Oncol 27:186-192
46. Quasar Collaborative G, Gray R, Barnwell J et al (2007) Adjuvant chemotherapy versus observation in patients with colorectal cancer: a randomised study. Lancet 370:2020-2029
47. Ribic CM, Sargent DJ, Moore MJ et al (2003) Tumor microsatellite-instability status as a predictor of benefit from fluorouracil-based adjuvant chemotherapy for colon cancer. N Engl J Med 349:247-257
48. Koopman M, Kortman GA, Mekenkamp L et al (2009) Deficient mismatch repair system in patients with sporadic advanced colorectal cancer. Br J Cancer 100:266-273
49. Sargent DJ, Marsoni S, Monges G et al (2010) Defective mismatch repair as a predictive marker for lack of efficacy of fluorouracil-based adjuvant therapy in colon cancer. J Clin Oncol 28:3219-3226

50. Benatti P, Gafa R, Barana D et al (2005) Microsatellite instability and colorectal cancer prognosis. Clin Cancer Res 11:8332-8340
51. Jover R, Zapater P, Castells A et al (2009) The efficacy of adjuvant chemotherapy with 5-fluorouracil in colorectal cancer depends on the mismatch repair status. Eur J Cancer 45:365-373
52. Bertagnolli MM, Niedzwiecki D, Compton CC et al (2009) Microsatellite instability predicts improved response to adjuvant therapy with irinotecan, fluorouracil, and leucovorin in stage III colon cancer: Cancer and Leukemia Group B Protocol 89803. J Clin Oncol 27:1814-1821
53. Fallik D, Borrini F, Boige V et al (2003) Microsatellite instability is a predictive factor of the tumor response to irinotecan in patients with advanced colorectal cancer. Cancer Res 63:5738-5744
54. Tejpar S, Bertagnolli M, Bosman F et al (2010) Prognostic and predictive biomarkers in resected colon cancer: current status and future perspectives for integrating genomics into biomarker discovery. Oncologist 15:390-404
55. Boulay JL, Mild G, Lowy A et al (2002) SMAD4 is a predictive marker for 5-fluorouracil-based chemotherapy in patients with colorectal cancer. Br J Cancer 87:630-634
56. Alhopuro P, Alazzouzi H, Sammalkorpi H et al (2005) SMAD4 levels and response to 5-fluorouracil in colorectal cancer. Clin Cancer Res 11:6311-6316
57. Tol J, Koopman M, Cats A et al (2009) Chemotherapy, bevacizumab, and cetuximab in metastatic colorectal cancer. N Engl J Med 360:563-572
58. Van Cutsem E, Kohne CH, Hitre E et al (2009) Cetuximab and chemotherapy as initial treatment for metastatic colorectal cancer. N Engl J Med 360:1408-1417
59. Overman MJ, Hoff PM (2007) EGFR-targeted therapies in colorectal cancer. Dis Colon Rectum 50:1259-1270
60. Moroni M, Veronese S, Benvenuti S et al (2005) Gene copy number for epidermal growth factor receptor (EGFR) and clinical response to antiEGFR treatment in colorectal cancer: a cohort study. Lancet Oncol 6:279-286
61. Normanno N, Tejpar S, Morgillo F (2009) Implications for KRAS status and EGFR-targeted therapies in metastatic CRC. Nat Rev Clin Oncol 6:519-527
62. Maestro ML, Vidaurreta M, Sanz-Casla MT et al (2007) Role of the BRAF mutations in the microsatellite instability genetic pathway in sporadic colorectal cancer. Ann Surg Oncol 14:1229-1236
63. Di Nicolantonio F, Martini M, Molinari F et al (2008) Wild-type BRAF is required for response to panitumumab or cetuximab in metastatic colorectal cancer. J Clin Oncol 26:5705-5712
64. Laurent-Puig P, Cayre A, Manceau G et al (2009) Analysis of PTEN, BRAF, and EGFR status in determining benefit from cetuximab therapy in wild-type KRAS metastatic colon cancer. J Clin Oncol 27:5924-5930
65. Sartore-Bianchi A, Di Nicolantonio F, Nichelatti M et al (2009) Multi-determinants analysis of molecular alterations for predicting clinical benefit to EGFR-targeted monoclonal antibodies in colorectal cancer. PLoS One 4:e7287
66. Bianco R, Shin I, Ritter CA et al (2003) Loss of PTEN/MMAC1/TEP in EGF receptor-expressing tumor cells counteracts the antitumor action of EGFR tyrosine kinase inhibitors. Oncogene 22:2812-2822
67. She Y, Lee F, Chen J et al (2003) The epidermal growth factor receptor tyrosine kinase inhibitor ZD1839 selectively potentiates radiation response of human tumors in nude mice, with a marked improvement in therapeutic index. Clin Cancer Res 9:3773-3778
68. Frattini M, Saletti P, Romagnani E et al (2007) PTEN loss of expression predicts cetuximab efficacy in metastatic colorectal cancer patients. Br J Cancer 97:1139-1145
69. Loupakis F, Pollina L, Stasi I et al (2009) PTEN expression and KRAS mutations on primary tumors and metastases in the prediction of benefit from cetuximab plus irinotecan for patients with metastatic colorectal cancer. J Clin Oncol 27:2622-2629
70. Russo A, Bazan V, Iacopetta B et al (2005) The TP53 colorectal cancer international collaborative study on the prognostic and predictive significance of p53 mutation: influence of tumor site, type of mutation, and adjuvant treatment. J Clin Oncol 23:7518-7528

71. Matlashewski GJ, Tuck S, Pim D et al (1987) Primary structure polymorphism at amino acid residue 72 of human p53. Mol Cell Biol 7:961-963
72. Tominaga T, Iwahashi M, Takifuji K et al (2010) Combination of p53 codon 72 polymorphism and inactive p53 mutation predicts chemosensitivity to 5-fluorouracil in colorectal cancer. Int J Cancer 126:1691-1701
73. Boneberg EM, Legler DF, Hoefer MM et al (2009) Angiogenesis and lymphangiogenesis are downregulated in primary breast cancer. Br J Cancer 101:605-614
74. Croner RS, Fortsch T, Bruckl WM et al (2008) Molecular signature for lymphatic metastasis in colorectal carcinomas. Ann Surg 247:803-810
75. Lu AT, Salpeter SR, Reeve AE et al(2009) Gene expression profiles as predictors of poor outcomes in stage II colorectal cancer: A systematic review and meta-analysis. Clin Colorectal Cancer 8:207-214
76. Garman KS, Acharya CR, Edelman E et al (2008) A genomic approach to colon cancer risk stratification yields biologic insights into therapeutic opportunities. Proc Natl Acad Sci U S A 105:19432-19437
77. Watanabe T, Kobunai T, Sakamoto E et al (2009) Gene expression signature for recurrence in stage III colorectal cancers. Cancer 115:283-292
78. Watanabe T, Wu TT, Catalano PJ et al (2001) Molecular predictors of survival after adjuvant chemotherapy for colon cancer. N Engl J Med 344:1196-1206
79. Ebert MP, Tanzer M, Balluff B et al (2012) TFAP2E-DKK4 and chemoresistance in colorectal cancer. N Engl J Med 366:44-53
80. Baker JB, Dutta D, Watson D et al (2011) Tumor gene expression predicts response to cetuximab in patients with KRAS wild-type metastatic colorectal cancer. Br J Cancer 104:488-495
81. Scartozzi M, Bearzi I, Mandolesi A et al (2011) Epidermal growth factor receptor (EGFR) gene promoter methylation and cetuximab treatment in colorectal cancer patients. Br J Cancer 104:1786-1790
82. Koukourakis MI, Giatromanolaki A, Sivridis E et al (2011) Prognostic and predictive role of lactate dehydrogenase 5 expression in colorectal cancer patients treated with PTK787/ZK 222584 (vatalanib) antiangiogenic therapy. Clin Cancer Res 17:4892-4900
83. Watanabe T, Kobunai T, Yamamoto Y et al (2011) Gene expression of vascular endothelial growth factor A, thymidylate synthase, and tissue inhibitor of metalloproteinase 3 in prediction of response to bevacizumab treatment in colorectal cancer patients. Dis Colon Rectum 54:1026-1035
84. Diasio RB, Johnson MR (2000) The role of pharmacogenetics and pharmacogenomics in cancer chemotherapy with 5-fluorouracil. Pharmacology 61:199-203
85. Wei X, McLeod HL, McMurrough J et al (1996) Molecular basis of the human dihydropyrimidine dehydrogenase deficiency and 5-fluorouracil toxicity. J Clin Invest 98:610-615
86. Cohen V, Panet-Raymond V, Sabbaghian N et al (2003) Methylenetetrahydrofolate reductase polymorphism in advanced colorectal cancer: a novel genomic predictor of clinical response to fluoropyrimidine-based chemotherapy. Clin Cancer Res 9:1611-1615
87. Lecomte T, Landi B, Beaune P et al (2006) Glutathione S-transferase P1 polymorphism (Ile105Val) predicts cumulative neuropathy in patients receiving oxaliplatin-based chemotherapy. Clin Cancer Res 12:3050-3056
88. Watson MA, Stewart RK, Smith GB et al (1998) Human glutathione S-transferase P1 polymorphisms: relationship to lung tissue enzyme activity and population frequency distribution. Carcinogenesis 19:275-280
89. McLeod HL, Sargent DJ, Marsh S et al (2010) Pharmacogenetic predictors of adverse events and response to chemotherapy in metastatic colorectal cancer: results from North American Gastrointestinal Intergroup Trial N9741. J Clin Oncol 28:3227-3233
90. Hoskins JM, Goldberg RM, Qu P et al (2007) UGT1A1*28 genotype and irinotecan-induced neutropenia: dose matters. J Natl Cancer Inst 99:1290-1295
91. Marsh S, McLeod HL (2001) Thymidylate synthase pharmacogenetics in colorectal cancer. Clin Colorectal Cancer 1:175-178

92. Bohanes P, Labonte MJ, Lenz HJ (2011) A review of excision repair cross-complementation group 1 in colorectal cancer. Clin Colorectal Cancer 10:157-164
93. Grimminger PP, Shi M, Barrett C et al (2011) TS and ERCC-1 mRNA expressions and clinical outcome in patients with metastatic colon cancer in CONFIRM-1 and -2 clinical trials. Pharmacogenomics J, in press
94. Spindler KL, Andersen RF, Jensen LH et al (2010) EGF61A>G polymorphism as predictive marker of clinical outcome to first-line capecitabine and oxaliplatin in metastatic colorectal cancer. Ann Oncol 21:535-539
95. Loupakis F, Ruzzo A, Salvatore L et al (2011) Retrospective exploratory analysis of VEGF polymorphisms in the prediction of benefit from first-line FOLFIRI plus bevacizumab in metastatic colorectal cancer. BMC Cancer 11:247
96. Murdoch C, Muthana M, Coffelt SB, Lewis CE (2008) The role of myeloid cells in the promotion of tumor angiogenesis. Nat Rev Cancer 8:618-631
97. Shojaei F, Wu X, Malik AK et al (2007) Tumor refractoriness to anti-VEGF treatment is mediated by CD11b+Gr1+ myeloid cells. Nat Biotechnol 25:911-920
98. Yang L, DeBusk LM, Fukuda K et al (2004) Expansion of myeloid immune suppressor Gr+CD11b+ cells in tumor-bearing host directly promotes tumor angiogenesis. Cancer Cell 6:409-421
99. Sakata K, Kwok TT, Murphy BJ et al (1991) Hypoxia-induced drug resistance: comparison to P-glycoprotein-associated drug resistance. Br J Cancer 64:809-814
100. Carmeliet P, Jain RK (2005) Principles and mechanisms of vessel normalization for cancer and other angiogenic diseases. Nat Rev Drug Discov 10:417-427
101. Jain RK (2005) Normalization of tumor vasculature: an emerging concept in antiangiogenic therapy. Science 307:58-62
102. Minoo P, Zlobec I, Peterson M et al (2010) Characterization of rectal, proximal and distal colon cancers based on clinicopathological, molecular and protein profiles. Int J Oncol 37:707-718
103. Slattery ML, Curtin K, Wolff RK et al (2009) A comparison of colon and rectal somatic DNA alterations. Dis Colon Rectum 52:1304-1311
104. Kalady MF, Sanchez JA, Manilich E et al (2009) Divergent oncogenic changes influence survival differences between colon and rectal adenocarcinomas. Dis Colon Rectum 52:1039-1045
105. Li JN, Zhao L, Wu J et al (2012) Differences in gene expression profiles and carcinogenesis pathways between colon and rectal cancer. J Dig Dis 13:24-32
106. Kapiteijn E, Liefers GJ, Los LC et al (2001) Mechanisms of oncogenesis in colon versus rectal cancer. J Pathol 195:171-178
107. Russo A, Bazan V, Iacopetta B et al (2005) The TP53 colorectal cancer international collaborative study on the prognostic and predictive significance of p53 mutation: influence of tumor site, type of mutation, and adjuvant treatment. J Clin Oncol 23:7518-7528
108. Birkenkamp-Demtroder K, Olesen SH, Sorensen FB et al (2005) Differential gene expression in colon cancer of the caecum versus the sigmoid and rectosigmoid. Gut 54:374-384
109. Fric P, Sovova V, Sloncova E et al (2009) Different expression of some molecular markers in sporadic cancer of the left and right colon. Eur J Cancer Prev 9:265-268

Neo- and Adjuvant Therapy

5

Alessandra Guglielmi

5.1 Introduction

The last two decades have witnessed the integration of a multimodality approach to locally advanced (≥ cT3 any N or any T N+) rectal cancers.

Improvements in preoperative staging with endorectal ultrasound and magnetic resonance imaging, the use of more accurate surgical techniques (total mesorectal excision) (TME), the wide use of preoperative or postoperative chemoradiation (CRT) have optimized local treatment and led to local failure rates of less than 10%.

The optimal sequence of surgery and chemoradiation has been addressed in several randomized trials, and preoperative modality has been shown to be superior to postoperative treatment.

The major advantages of preoperative treatment are: 1) tumor down-staging, with increased resectability, higher probability of obtaining tumor-free circumferential resection margins (CRM) and, in some cases, sphincter preservation; 2) reduced incidence of acute and chronic toxicity; 3) improved systemic control on micrometastases.

Table 5.1 shows a selection of published and ongoing "paradigm changing" trials in the treatment of rectal cancer.

In 1997 the Swedish Rectal Cancer Trial produced evidence that preoperative short-course radiotherapy (RT) (25 Gy in 5 daily/fractions, followed by surgery after 1-week rest) reduces the risk of local recurrence (11% vs. 27% with surgery alone). Unfortunately the improvement in median overall survival (OS) observed in this study has not been confirmed in subsequent trials [1, 2].

A. Guglielmi (✉)
Department of Oncology, "Ospedali Riuniti" University Hospital,
Trieste, Italy
e-mail: alessandra.guglielmi@aots.sanita.fvg.it

N. de Manzini (ed.), *Rectal Cancer*,
Updates in Surgery
DOI: 10.1007/978-88-470-2670-4_5,

Table 5.1 Randomized trials comparing dose and timing of RT and surgery in locally advanced rectal cancer

Trial (year)	Patient's number	Follow-up (months)	Treatment design	Local recurrence	Overall survival
Swedish Rectal Cancer Trial (1997) [1]	1168	60	Neoadjuvant short-course RT vs surgery	11% vs. 27% ($p<0.001$)	58% vs. 48% ($p=0.004$)
Dutch TME trial (2001) [3]	1861	24	Neoadjuvant short-course RT + surgery (standard TME) vs. surgery alone (standard TME)	2.4% vs. 8.2% ($p<0.001$)	82% vs. 81.8% ($p=0.84$)
German Rectal Cancer Study Group (CAO/ARO/AIO-94) (2004) (2011) [4, 5]	799	120	Neoadjuvant long-course RT +CT *vs* adjuvant long-course RT+CT	5.7% vs. 10.4% ($p=0.009$)	59.9% v.s 59.5% ($p=0.86$)
NSABP R-03 (2009) [6]	254	60	Neoadjuvant long-course RT+CT vs postoperative long-course RT+CT	10.7% vs. 10.7% ($p=0.69$)	74.5% vs. 65.6% ($p=0.065$)
Stockholm III (2010) [7]	303	ongoing	Neoadjuvant short-course RT + surgery within 1 wk vs. neoadjuvant short-course + surgery 4 to 8 wk later vs. neoadjuvant long-course RT + surgery 4 to 8 wk later	ongoing	ongoing

CAO/ARO/AIO, Chirurgische Arbeitsgemeinschaft für Onkologie/ Arbeitsgemeinschaft Radiologische Onkologie / Arbeitsgemeinschaft Internistische Onkologie; *NSABP*, National Surgical Adjuvant Breast and Bowel Project; *ECOG*, Eastern Cooperative Oncology Group; *CT*, chemotherapy

The introduction in clinical practice of standard TME in 2001 reduced the risk of local relapse. The benefits of TME are increased by the preoperative use of short-course radiotherapy (RT): local relapse rates are 8.2% with TME alone vs. 2.4% with TME +RT, (p <0.001). These results emphasize the importance of obtaining negative CRM and the effect of preoperative treatments on T4 tumor down-staging, enhancing surgeon performance [3].

Along the same lines, fluoropyrimidine-based chemotherapy in addition to preoperative or postoperative long-course RT (45-50.4 Gy administered over 5-6 weeks, followed by surgery after a period of 6-8 weeks rest) was explored in two large randomized trials: the "German study" and the NSABP-R03.

The German study (CAO/ARO/AIO-94) shows, with an accrual of 799 eligible patients, that the preoperative approach is superior to the postoperative one in terms of: 1) local control (6% vs. 13%, p=0.006); 2) acute toxic effects (27 vs. 40% , p=0.001), 3) chronic toxic effects (14 vs. 24%, p=0.012). Sphincter preservation, in patients judged by the surgeon to require an abdominoperineal approach, is also improved with preoperative CRT (39 vs. 19%, p=0.005) [4]. At the ASCO meeting last year the 10-year follow-up data were presented (Table 5.1), and confirmed that local control is better with the preoperative approach. Unfortunately, this result did not translate into an OS advantage [5].

The NSABP R-03 trial was closed prematurely because of poor patient accrual, but the results have been recently reported for 254 (of 900 scheduled) patients after a median follow-up of 8.4 years. The 5-year disease-free survival (DFS) in this trial was significantly improved for patients treated with preoperative rather than postoperative therapy (65% vs. 53% p=0.011). The increase in 5-year OS, although not statistically significant, was 75% vs. 66% for patients treated pre- and postoperatively, respectively (p=0.065). Both regimens were effective in terms of reduction of local recurrence (10.7 % in both arms) [6].

An important issue, regarding the optimal schedule of RT and the interval between the end of treatment and surgery, is under investigation by the Stockholm III study. In this trial patients with resectable rectal cancers were randomized to receive neoadjuvant short-course RT, followed by immediate or delayed (4-8 weeks later) surgery, vs. neoadjuvant long-course RT followed by surgery, 4-8 weeks later. The interim analysis, published in 2010, showed similar results for the three arms in terms of feasibility, acute toxicity and perioperative complications. Delayed surgery increases the down-staging effect in both short- and long-course RT [7]. These data are particularly interesting for their future implications in some clinical conditions e.g., elderly patients with operable locally advanced rectal tumors, unable to tolerate long-course treatment.

In addition, two large, randomized trials published in recent years (not reported in Table 5.1) explored whether CRT is more convenient than RT alone in the preoperative setting and the role of postoperative chemotherapy (4 cycles) in patients with T3-T4 or N+ rectal cancer.

The European Organization for Research and Treatment of Cancer 22921 is a four arm trial comparing preoperative RT (45Gy) with or without bolus fluorouracil/leucovorin, followed by surgery, with or without 4 cycles of adjuvant chemotherapy. A significant decrease in local recurrence was observed in the three chemotherapy groups: 8.8%, 9.6%, 8.0% with either preoperative CRT, postoperative CT or both, respectively, compared with 17.1% with RT alone.

The addition of chemotherapy did not affect the 5-year OS at a median follow-up of 5.4 years (65.6% vs. 64.8% $p=0.79$) for CRT vs. RT alone, and 67% vs. 63% for adjuvant CT vs. no adjuvant treatment [8].

The second trial was conducted by the Féderation Francophone de Cancérologie Digestive (FFCD) 9203, comparing preoperative RT (45Gy) with or without bolus fluorouracil/leucovorin. All patients received four cycles of chemotherapy with the same regimen in the postoperative setting. In this trial the rate of pathological complete responses (pCR) (11.4% vs. 3.6% $p=0.0001$), and the lower percentage of local recurrences (8.1% vs. 16.5%, $p=0.004$) are in favor of preoperative CRT. No differences in 5-yr OS were observed between arms [9].

Given all these data, fluoropyrimidine-based (bolus or continuous infusion) preoperative CRT followed by four cycles of adjuvant fluorouracil-based chemotherapy is the preferred treatment for patients with locally advanced rectal cancer. A total of approximately six months of perioperative treatment is preferred.

The oral fluorouracil pro-drug Capecitabine is nowadays largely accepted as a substitute for fluorouracil in the neoadjuvant setting due to its advantageous safety profile, improved nodal down-staging and favorable survival data [10].

Postoperative treatment for a total of 6 months combining chemo (fluorouracil-based) and radiotherapy should always be given in the case of upfront surgery in patients with:1) involved CRM; 2) perforation in the tumor area; and 3) pT ≥3 and/ or pN+ tumors.

The interval between surgery and the start of adjuvant chemotherapy is very important. A recent meta-analysis of 10 studies involving more than 15,000 patients with colorectal cancer showed that each 4-week delay results in a 14% decrease in OS, indicating that chemotherapy should be started as soon as the patient is medically able to tolerate it [11].

5.2 Integrating New Drugs in Combined Modality of Neoadjuvant and Adjuvant Treatment of Rectal Cancer

5.2.1 Chemotherapy

The positive correlation between pathologic stage and disease free-survival after neoadjuvant CRT, and the knowledge that development of distant metastases is the predominant mode of failure in rectal cancer (30 to 35%), justify the attempt to use more active agents in combination with RT, in order to increase the percentage of response rates, prolong DFS and, possibly, OS.

A combination of newer chemotherapy drugs, such as oral fluropyrimidines, oxaliplatin and irinotecan, has been incorporated in phase I and II trials. Most of these studies result in higher pCR rates at the cost of higher, but manageable, toxicity.

Table 5.2 reports the published phase III studies exploring the effect of oral fluoropyrimidines and oxaliplatin in the neo-adjuvant setting. So far no data are available on DFS and OS, but pathologic complete responses are not statistically different between experimental and control arm in both trials, whereas the co-administration of fluoropyrimidine and oxaliplatin results in increased acute grade 3-4 toxicity [12, 13]. Aschele and co-authors conclude that "these data argue against the use of oxaliplatin/fluorouracil/RT as a platform for the incorporation of biologic agents in the treatment of this disease in order to ameliorate the results of pre-operative CRT".

Table 5.3 lists the ongoing phase III trials exploring different doses of RT, different schedules of fluoropyrimidine (oral, prolonged i.v. or bolus) and less or more intensive adjuvant treatments (fluroropyrimidine ±oxaliplatin ± biologic agents). The results of these studies could mean an improvement over the next few years of the optimal combined treatment for locally advanced rectal cancer.

5.2.2 Biological Agents

According to results obtained in the treatment of advanced colorectal cancers, both Avastin (an anti-vascular endothelial growth-factor) and Erbitux (an inhibitor of the epidermal growth factor receptor) have been employed in combination with CRT in phase I and II studies. Despite positive preclinical data the results obtained with Erbitux have been disappointing, in phase II studies, in terms of low pCR rates [14-16].

The data observed with Avastin are more intriguing: higher pCR rates with Avastin, fluorouracil and RT, but a word of caution is mandatory for the toxicity pattern (radiation induced enteritis, perforations) and surgical complications (wound healing, fistula, bleeding) [17].

For these reasons there is no indication for their use in clinical practice.

The real challenge, for the near future, is patient selection according to molecular markers (EGFR gene copy number, mutational status of K-RAS, B-RAF, etc). The possibility of identifying patients with responsive tumors at the time of diagnosis should lead to a selective, personalized approach, avoiding toxicity and, in selected cases, more radical surgery.

Table 5.2 Published Phase III trials with new agents in locally advanced rectal cancer

Trial (year)	Patient's number	Surgery	Treatment design	Adjuvant	Primary endpoint	%pCR	Toxicity grade ≥ 3
ACCORD 12/0405 (2010) [12]	598	TME	RT 45 Gy + CAPE vs RT 45 Gy + CAPE +Ox	CT free in each center	% of pCR	13.9 vs. 19.2 P= NS	11% vs. 25%
STAR-01 (2011) [13]	747	TME	RT 45 Gy + FU PVI vs RT 45 Gy + FU PVI+ Weekly Ox	fluorouracil-based CT	DFS	16% in both arms	8% vs 24%

FU, 5-fluorouracil; *Ox*, Oxaliplatin; *CAPE*, Capecitabine; *PVI*, Protracted Venous Infusion; *ACCORD*, Actions Concertées dans les Cancers Colorectaux et Digestifs; *STAR*, Studio nazionale Terapia neoAdiuvante Retto

Table 5.3 Ongoing Phase III trials with new chemotherapeutic agents in locally advanced rectal cancer

Trial (year)	Surgery	Treatment design	Adjuvant	Primary endpoint	Status
NSABP R-04 (2011) [18]	TME	RT 50.4 Gy + FU vs. RT 50.4 Gy + FU+ Ox vs. RT 50.4 Gy + CAPE vs. RT 50.4 Gy + CAPE+ Ox	FOLFOX vs. FOLFOX + Avastin	loco-regional relapse rate	follow-up
ECOG-E5204	TME	RT 40-55.8 Gy + chemotherapy according to NSABP R-04 or FU PVI/CAPE ±OX or FU/LV	FOLFOX vs. FOLFOX +Avastin	overall survival	stopped
CAO/ARO/AIO-04 (2011) [19]	TME	RT 50.4 Gy + FU vs. RT 50.4 Gy + FU +Ox	FU vs. FU + Ox	disease-free survival	follow-up
PETACC-6	TME	RT 45 Gy + CAPE vs. RT 45 Gy +CAPE+ Ox	CAPE vs. CAPE + Ox	disease-free survival	follow-up

NSABP, National Surgical Adjuvant Breast and Bowel Project; *ECOG*, Eastern Cooperative Oncology Group; *CAO/ARO/AIO*, Chirurgische Arbeitsgemeinschaft für Onkologie/ Arbeitsgemeinschaft Radiologische Onkologie / Arbeitsgemeinschaft Internistische Onkologie; *PETACC*, Pan-European Trials in Alimentary Tract Cancer; *FU*, 5-fluorouracil; *Ox*, Oxaliplatin; *CAPE*, Capecitabine; *PVI*, protracted venous infusion; *LV*, leucovorin

5.3 Palliative Therapy (Stage IV at Diagnosis)

Approximately 20% of patients with rectal cancer have metastases at diagnosis. The approach to these patients is always multidisciplinary and is guided by: 1) tumor burden, local and at distance; 2) presence of rectal symptoms (bleeding, obstruction, pain); 3) age and comorbidities; 4) molecular determinants (K-RAS and B-RAF mutational status). Figure 5.1 outlines possible scenarios and offers some indications for this subset of patients.

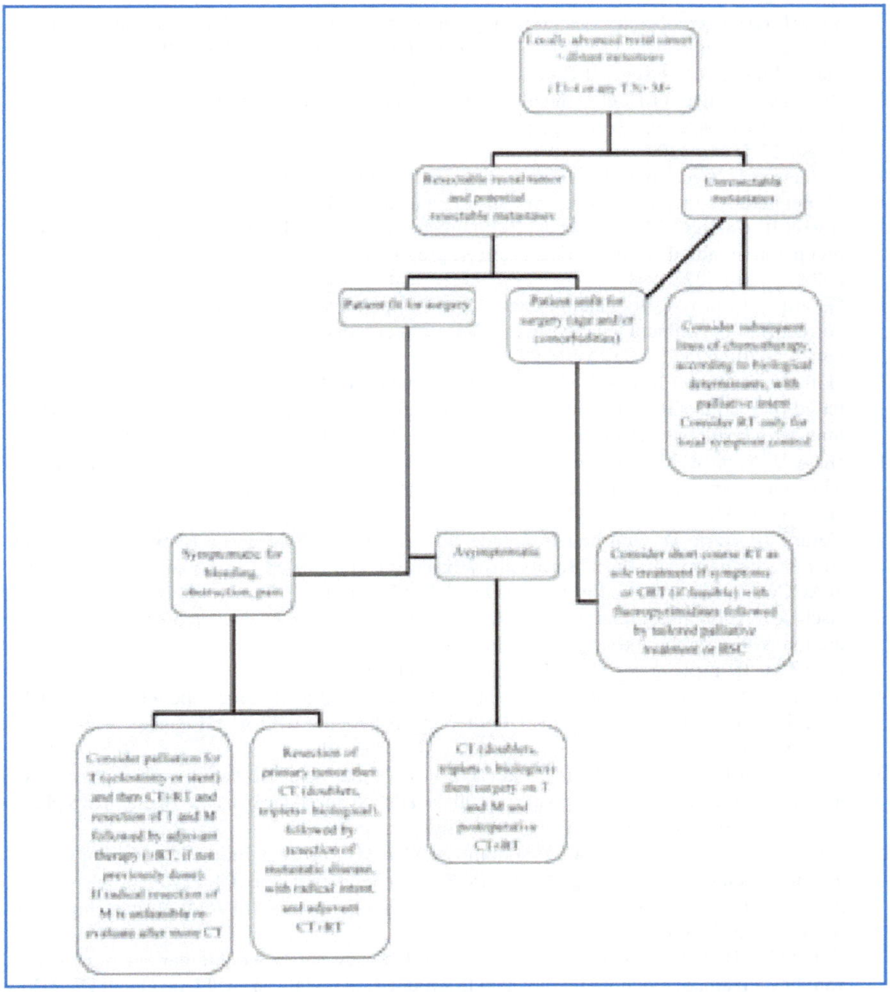

Fig. 5.1 Doublets: FOLFIRI, FOLFOX, XELOX; triplets: FOLFOXIRI; *BSC*, best supportive care; *T*, primary tumor; *M*, metastases

References

1. Improved survival with preoperative radiotherapy in resectable rectal cancer. Swedish Rectal Cancer Trial (1997) N Engl J Med 336: 980-987
2. Bujko K, Nowacki MP, Nasierowska-Guttmejer A et al (2006) Long-term results of a randomized trial comparing preoperative short-course radiotherapy with preoperative conventionally fractionated chemoradiation for rectal cancer. Br J Surg 93:1215-1223
3. Kapiteijn E, Marijnen CA, Nagtegaal ID et al (2001) Preoperative radiotherapy combined with total mesorectal excision for resectable rectal cancer. N Engl J Med 345:638-646
4. Sauer R, Becker H, Hohenberger P et al (2004) Preoperative chemoradiotherapy as compared with postoperative chemoradiotherapy for locally advanced rectal cancer. N Engl J Med 351:11-20
5. Sauer R (2011) Preoperative versus postoperative chemoradiotherapy for locally advanced rectal cancer: results of the German CAO/ARO/AIO-94 randomized phase III trial after a median follow-up of 11 years. J Clin Oncol 29 (suppl) abs 3516
6. Roh MS, Colangelo LH, O'Connell MJ et al (2009) Preoperative multimodality therapy improves disease-free survival in patients with carcinoma of the rectum: NSABP R-03. J Clin Oncol 27:5124-5130
7. Pettersson D, Cedermark B, Holm T et al (2010) Interim analysis of the Stockholm III trial of preoperative radiotherapy regimens for rectal cancer. Br J Surg 97:580-587
8. Bosset JF, Calais G, Mineur L et al (2005) Enhanced tumorocidal effect of chemotherapy with preoperative radiotherapy for rectal cancer: preliminary results—EORTC 22921. J Clin Oncol 23:5620-5627
9. Gerard JP, Conroy T, Bonnetain F et al (2006) Preoperative radiotherapy with or without concurrent fluorouracil and leucovorin in T3-4 rectal cancers: results of FFCD 9203. J Clin Oncol 24:4620-4625
10. Hofheinz R, Wenz FK, Post S et al (2011) Capecitabine (CAPE) versus 5-Fluorouracil (5-FU)-based (neo)adjuvant chemoradiotherapy (CRT) for locally advanced rectal cancer (LARC): long-term results of a randomized phase III trial. J Clin Oncol 29 (suppl) abs 3504
11. Biagi JJ, Raphael MJ, Mackillop WJ et al (2011) Association between time to initiation of adjuvant chemotherapy and survival in colorectal cancer: a systematic review and meta-analysis. JAMA 305:2335-2342
12. Gerard JP, Azria D, Gourgou-Bourgade S et al (2010) Comparison of two neoadjuvant chemoradiotherapy regimens for locally advanced rectal cancer. Results of the phase III trial ACCORD 12/0405-Prodige. J Clin Oncol 28:1638-1644
13. Aschele C, Cionini L, Lonardi S et al (2011) Primary tumor response to preoperative chemoradiation with or without oxaliplatin in locally advanced rectal cancer: pathological results of the STAR-01 randomized phase III trial. J Clin Oncol 29:2773-2780
14. Machiels JP, Sempoux C, Scalliet P et al (2007) Phase I/II study of preoperative cetuximab, capecitabine, and external beam radiotherapy in patients with rectal cancer. Ann Oncol 18:738-744
15. Horisberger K, Treschl A, Mai S et al (2009) Cetuximab in combination with capecitabine, irinotecan , and radiotherapy for patients with locally advanced rectal cancer. Results of a phase II MARGIT trial. Int J Radiat Oncol Biol Phys 74:1487-1493
16. Dewdney A (2011) EXPERT-C:A randomized, phase II European multicenter trial of neoadjuvant capecitabine plus oxaliplatin (CAPOX) and chemo radiation (CRT) with or without cetuximab followed by total mesorectal excision (TME) in patients with RMI-defined, high-risk rectal cancer. J Clin Oncol 29 (suppl) abs 3513
17. Willet CG, Duda DG, di Tomaso E et al (2009) Efficacy, safety and biomarkers of neoadjuvant bevacizumab, radiation therapy and fluorouracil in rectal cancer. J Clin Oncol 27:3020-3026
18. Roh MS (2011) The impact of capecitabine and oxaliplatin in the preoperative multimodality treatment in patients with carcinoma of the rectum: NSABP R-04. J Clin Oncol 29 (suppl) abs 3503

19. Roedel C (2011) Preoperative chemoradiotherapy and postoperative chemotherapy with 5-fluorouracil and oxaliplatin versus 5-fluorouracil alone in locally advanced rectal cancer. First results of the German CAO/ARO/AIO-04 randomized phase III study. J Clin Oncol 29 (suppl) abs 3505

Perioperative Treatment

6

Biagio Casagranda, Roberta Cavallin and Nicolò de Manzini

6.1 Introduction

Perioperative management in patients who are to undergo a surgical operation is extremely important to achieve the optimum outcome of surgery.

The effective reduction of postoperative mortality and postoperative morbidity for all age classes is connected to improvements in surgical and anesthesiology techniques as well as in advanced perioperative management (Fast-Track) [1].

Perioperative activity can be broken down into procedures carried out:

- before the operation (intestinal preparation, pre-operative nutrition, antibiotic prophylaxis, antithrombotic prophylaxis, bladder catheter);
- during the operation (insertion of nasogastric probe (NGP), fluid therapy, abdominal drainage);
- after the operation (early oral feeding, NRS pain control (Numeric Pain Intensity Scale), early mobilization).

Improvements in perioperative activity have meant a reduction of hospitalization and with it an improvement in the outcome of the patient, guaranteeing a lower degree of operative and preoperative stress, excellent pain control, and a reduction in organ dysfunction, as well as a saving of hospital resources [2].

In this connection, a single "Fast Track" surgery programme called ERAS (Enhanced Recovery After Surgery) has recently been drawn up, combining several protocols for patients undergoing colorectal surgery [3]. The protocol envisages: no intestinal preparation or pre-medication, the use of epidural

B. Casagranda (✉)
Department of Medicine, Surgery and Health Sciences, General Surgery Unit,
Cattinara University Hospital,
Trieste, Italy
e-mail: biagio.casagranda@aots.sanita.fvg.it

N. de Manzini (ed.), *Rectal Cancer,*
Updates in Surgery
DOI: 10.1007/978-88-470-2670-4_6,

anesthesia for perioperative analgesia, carbohydrate-rich liquids up to 2-3 hours prior to the operation, postoperative oxygen therapy, restriction of the infusion of fluids in the immediate postoperative period (6 ml/kg/h), non-routine use of NGP and abdominal drainage, early feeding and mobilization, respiratory physiotherapy [4, 5].

All this is designed to reduce complications (medical and surgical), bring forward oral food consumption, reduce the duration of ileus and early motor restoration, and as a consequence, reduce hospital stay and costs.

6.2 Intestinal Preparation

The classical approach to a colorectal operation envisages cleaning the intestine as completely as possible by using Mechanical Bowel Preparation (MBP). The total removal of the contents of the intestine, which is full of bacteria, is achieved by eliminating the feces.

One of the purposes of this manoeuvre is to reduce the possible complications involving infection (anastomotic leakage, peritonitis, septic shock, wall abscess, evisceration) [6].

Other theoretical advantages are: reducing contamination of the abdominal cavity and wall in the event of voluntary or accidental opening of the digestive tract; allowing easy manipulation of the emptied small intestine or colon; avoiding distension of a colic or colorectal anastomosis with passage of formed stool; allowing a quicker restoration of transit, because an empty colon contracts better than a colon and rectum full of feces; and limiting contamination in the event of leakage [7].

The patient is therefore informed about the procedure of the mechanical preparation (MBP), which is often difficult to perform because of concomitant collateral effects (nausea, vomit and dehydration), about the need for the help of health professionals or family members, and about the fact that it is not always possible to complete the procedure [6].

The MBP consists of taking: osmotic laxatives (Polyethylene Glycol, sodium dihydregen phosphate), which are the most used; saline laxatives (Sodium phosphate bisacodyl); stimulating laxatives; and anthracene purgatives (Sennoside B); mannitol and lactated Ringer's solution are also used (some protocols may require a combined approach).

Most of the studies performed in the last few decades suggest polyethylene glycol (PEG), 4 litres, as the best classic preparation for flushing the colon, both as regards cleaning and in terms of infective complications [7]. However, it has been observed that this kind of preparation may cause greater distension of the ileal loops, making it more difficult to see the colon-rectum during laparoscopy.

Recent studies have demonstrated that patients not subjected to mechanical preparation have a faster resumption of intestinal functions than those undergoing MBP; however, mechanical preparation is considered necessary in selected cases requiring intraoperative colonoscopy [3].

MBP does not reduce any complications due to colic surgery; it may even be the cause of inflammation of the mucosa, with a consequent progressive lesion and increase in mucus production, with resulting dysfunction of the intestinal wall [6].

A recent trial, GRECCAR III, carried out by a French multi-centre group (Bretagnol F, Panis Y et al.), compared 178 patients subjected to rectal resection: 89 prepared with the use of oral laxatives and enemas and 89 without any MBP. This study highlighted that the patients with MBP had a significantly lower rate of infection than those without preparation (27% vs. 44%, $p=0.018$). The differences in terms of anastomotic leakage, greater morbidity, postoperative hospitalization or mortality between the groups were not significant. The group therefore concluded by recommending mechanical preparation for rectal surgery [8].

A review by Cochrane in 2011 analysed 18 different trials, for a total of 5,805 patients put forward for elective colorectal surgery, divided into 2,906 subjected to MBP and 2,899 with no preparation.

This study revealed no statistically significant advantage between prepared patients and non-prepared patients in terms of morbidity, infections, anastomotic leakage and mortality [9].

It also confirmed that mechanical preparation is essential in patients requiring intraoperative colonoscopy, or to localise very small lesions in doubtful places [9, 10].

In our personal experience, all patients elected for rectal surgery are prescribed a low-residue diet for 7 days before the operation, along with probiotics and two low-pressure enemas performed the afternoon and the evening before surgery.

6.3 Anesthesia

Peri- and post-operative anesthesia and analgesia are essential for the early recovery of a patient undergoing an anterior resection of the rectum for cancer.

6.3.1 Pre-anesthetic Medication

Negative consequences deriving from the long-lasting effect of the premedication drugs used (opioids, sedatives with a long biological half-life, hypnotics) can hinder the recovery of the patient and prolong hospitalization. In this connection, the new anesthetic protocols do not envisage pre-anesthesia, but only an association between general and epidural anesthesia (there is no evidence that intraoperative epidural catheter analgesia can improve postoperative recovery, but its use has been observed to reduce the dosage of anesthetic used in general anesthesia). This eliminates the need to administer medicine like benzodiazepine, hitherto regarded as essential to sedate the patient before surgery .

Short duration anesthesia by inhalation was shown to be an excellent alternative for reducing the use of intravenous anesthesia and ensure a better postoperative course [3].

6.3.2 Managing Infusion Therapy in the Perioperative Period

In recent years the intravenous infusion of volumes of liquid greater than those effectively lost during the perioperative period has become standard practice.

The management of liquids in the perioperative period is still a controversial matter.

Traditional perioperative intravenous fluid regimens in abdominal surgery can lead to patients receiving 3.5 to 7 l of fluid on the day of surgery and more than 3 l/d for the following 3 to 4 days.

These rates can delay the return of normal gastrointestinal functioning, jeopardize healing of wounds or colorectal anastomosis, alter the effect of tissue oxygenation, or change heart and kidney function due to liquids leaking from vessels, with a consequent extension of the hospital stay. Some randomized controlled studies have demonstrated a reduction of morbidity and hospitalization in patients undergoing major surgery when the liquid infusion was set to achieve the optimum volume on the basis of a trans-esophageal echocardiogram (goal-directed fluid therapy) performed before or during the surgical operation.

Therefore, the best way to limit intravenous administration of liquids in the postoperative period is to stop intravenous infusions, with an early return to oral fluids, if possible as early as the first day after the operation [3].

6.3.3 Postoperative Analgesia

Good pain control after anterior resection of the rectum allows early mobilization of the patient.

Current pain treatment regimens consist of a combination of opioids or non-steroid inflammatory medication administered via epidural catheter. Furthermore, in the last ten years administration of local anesthetic in the wound has contributed to good pain control. In an elective anterior resection operation of the rectum, the epidural catheter is inserted into the thorax between T9-10, in the operating theatre and with the patient awake to avoid neurological complications. It is kept in place for 48-72 hours and permits a continual infusion of pain killers (local anesthetics). Studies have demonstrated that its use is correlated to a lower complication rate for the respiratory system and a quicker recovery of intestinal transit.

In the postoperative period, the use of opioids should be restricted due to their significant collateral effects, including nausea, vomiting and slowing of intestinal transit. Supportive therapies (e.g. antiemetics) to relieve the side effects of these drugs are in fact often required.

The use of non-steroid anti-inflammatory medication, or paracetamol, which has been seen to be effective in pain control, should be preferred [3]. However, a recent study published in the British Journal of Clinical Pharmacology highlights the hidden risks of using this pain killer. The team, made up of experts from the University of Edinburgh and the Scottish unit for liver transplants in Edinburgh, United Kingdom, stated that taking more paracetamol than necessary in the event of pain can cause an overdose. The conclusions of the team are based on an analysis of the data from 663 patients who had been hospitalized at the Royal Infirmary of Edinburgh between 1992 and 2008 with liver damage caused by paracetamol; 161 had taken an overdose. This means that almost one in four patients hospitalized with liver failure caused by paracetamol had accidentally taken an overdose of the medicine. This medication should therefore be used with great care, avoiding useless or even damaging overdoses [11].

The body's response to pain consists of the sum of the changes to the endocrine and metabolic system which can cause a slowing of the patient's recovery; if we add an anxiety-inducing element to this, the clinical picture will be rendered more complex, with a consequent further delay in the discharge of the patient .

6.4 Antithrombotic Prophylaxis

In abdominal surgery, the greatest risk of distal venous thrombosis assessed by paraclinical examination varies between 20 and 40%, and that of proximal venous thrombosis between 3 and 8%. The incidence of pulmonary embolism is 1.5-4% and in between 0.4 and 1% of cases it can lead to death.

In oncological surgery, the global risk of thrombotic events assessed through diagnostic exams is 30%, reaching 35% in colorectal surgery and 45% in cancer surgery of the small pelvis [7].

The thrombotic risk factors typical of these patients are:

- immobility, confinement to bed and paralysis of limbs;
- neoplasia and treatment of neoplasia (hormonal, chemotherapy, radiotherapy);
- previous thromboembolic events;
- age above 40;
- oral contraception with estrogens or hormone replacement therapy;
- heart and lung failure;
- inflammatory diseases of the intestine;
- myeloproliferative syndrome;
- obesity (BMI > 30);
- smoking;

- CVC (central venous catheter);
- acquired congenital thrombophilia.

Antithrombotic prophylaxis in colorectal surgery is performed with low molecular weight heparin administered subcutaneously (aspirin and K antivitamins are not recommended in this case). Studies have demonstrated that the duration of prevention is seven-ten days after digestive surgery, but longer-lasting treatment has been studied and recommended for major cancer surgery; in fact, by extending the prophylaxis to four weeks, paraclinical thrombosis is reduced by 50% without increasing the risk of hemorrhage [7, 12].

Elastic compression is recommended in the event of there being contra-indications to anticoagulant treatment and in association with pharmacological treatment, because it reduces the occurrence of paraclinical thromboembolic events by 66% in general surgery compared to no compression, and by 72% when used along with heparin compared to heparin alone.

Intermittent pneumatic compression complements pharmacological prophylaxis.

Prophylaxis with low molecular weight heparin must not be performed or must be suspended 12 hours before inserting or removing the epidural catheter [3].

6.5 Antibiotic Prophylaxis

Surgery of the digestive tract and/or its annexes may be clean (Altemeier class 1), if the digestive tract is not opened, or, as is usually the case, clean-contaminated (class 2), when the digestive tract is opened.

Rectal surgery therefore requires antibiotic-prophylaxis directed to a specific bacterial target, which is usually acknowledged as the main cause of post-surgery infections (e.g., Gram negative, Escherichia coli, Enterococcus and anaerobic bacteria) [7].

Antibiotic prophylaxis of elective rectal surgery usually consists of endovenous administration of second-generation cefalosporin (88% of cases) or amoxicillin with clavulanic acid (10% of cases); often either antibiotic may be associated with metronidazole. These therapies must be infused 30-60 minutes before the surgical incision (according to recent studies this occurs in 70% of cases) and continued for 24 hours after the operation [13].

The first dose administered is normally twice the usual one, because it is essential to maintain effective tissue rates or dosages indicated by the MIC, until the moment of closure. If surgery lasts longer than expected, re-infusions must be given during the operation at half the dose of the primary one.

The purpose of antibiotic prophylaxis is that of reducing wound infections, which usually represent 38% of the complications caused by colorectal surgery (and 17% of hospital-acquired infections), and of reducing general infections, if the contents of the digestive tract are disseminated. In the event of generalized infection, the prophylaxis may be changed to antibiotic therapy, in this case naturally by changing the antibiotic. The categories of patients at risk of wound infection, who may require a higher dose of antibiotic, are those affected by diabetes mellitus, those with stomy, or the elderly [14].

Protocols of antibiotic prophylaxis are established locally on the basis of the local bacterial epidemiology and of the cost/benefit ratio. Their effectiveness must be periodically reassessed and the protocols diversified according to the operation and the physiopathological characteristics of the patient undergoing surgery. Alternatives to antibiotic treatment must also be considered if the patient is allergic to the first choice molecule.

6.6 Nutrition

Under-nourishment is an important factor in morbidity and mortality, directly related to the duration of the hospital stay [12]. Early re-feeding makes it possible to limit postoperative under-nourishment, to improve immune functions, to reduce inflammatory response and to limit the permeability of the digestive wall, the source of bacterial translocation [7].

There are two different guidelines which can be referred to for a correct assessment of the nutritional state of the patient at the moment of hospitalization: ESPEN (European Clinical Nutrition and Metabolism) or ASPEN (American Society for Parenteral and Enteral Nutrition) [15, 16].

6.6.1 Preoperative Nutrition

Standard artificial preoperative nutrition is useless in those patients who are "slightly undernourished" and who can follow a nourishment programme that covers 60% of their needs.

Malnutrition particularly affects patients with neoplasia of the supramesocolic organs (esophagus, stomach) rather than the submesocolic ones.

In spite of this, patients with rectal neoplasia have a greater risk of malnutrition after neoadjuvant therapy, so it is recommended to carry out nutritional screening before the operation. Indeed, in the event of severe preoperative malnutrition, total parenteral nutrition is necessary to increase the protein intake, maintain muscle tone and preserve the cognitive and immune functions that are essential for a better patient outcome [5, 16].

6.6.2 Postoperative Nutrition

In the past, after major surgery, a long period of fasting was indicated followed by the administration of a liquid diet which did not change until a complete return to normal bowel function (only after the bowel opened to feces was a solid diet restored). Many surgeons agree that a liquid diet should be started 24 hours after surgery, whereas a return to feeding should begin after 48 hours or after the bowel has opened to gases and feces; this is due to the risk of anastomotic dehiscence or the onset of nausea and vomit, which would require the repositioning of an NGP for fear of Mendelson's syndrome.

Randomized prospective studies have demonstrated that early feeding reduces the onset of postoperative ileus and improves the immune functions, leading to a decrease in mortality and morbidity. However, to guarantee a quick return to feeding, there must be good control of postoperative nausea and vomiting , which often cause a delay in resuming oral intake.

The use of the following types of medication is therefore justified: 1) prokinetic agents, which stimulate gastrointestinal motility (e.g. Metoclopramide); 2) opiate antagonists (e.g. Naloxone) for bones, useful for restoring peristalsis; 3) antiemetics (e.g. Ondansetron), which reduce the onset of nausea and vomiting.

In conclusion, restoring early feeding does not significantly increase anastomotic dehiscence, infections or mortality rates.

Studies carried out on animal and human models have demonstrated that postoperative hyperglycemia is the cause of insulin resistance, which occurs as a reaction to various kinds of surgical aggression or stress, and does not help postoperative recovery.

Glucose passes from the blood to the hepatic cells by a difference in concentration, which is maintained by the transformation of the glucose into glucose-6-phosphate; in normoglycemia conditions this transformation is catalyzed by hexokinase, which is a slow enzyme, and by glucokinase, a fast enzyme which is activated when the insulin increases. The transformation into glycogen through other metabolic stages means that the reactions are not interrupted, thus allowing a further passage of glucose from the blood to the liver. An alteration of this complex biological system, called the Krebs cycle, may cause insulin resistance. This resistance may be reduced if preoperative fasting is replaced by an overload of carbohydrates taken orally or endovenously, and may be improved by providing a greater intake of glucose in the postoperative period [15].

Artificial postoperative nutrition is recommended in patients who:

- have received artificial preoperative nutrition;
- have not received artificial preoperative nutrition and who suffer from serious malnutrition;
- are incapable of taking food which covers 60% of their nutritional requirements within a week of the operation;
- present early postoperative complications responsible for an increase in metabolism and a longer period of fasting [7].

6.7 Nasogastric Probe (NGP)

Abdominal surgeons have used digestive aspiration with NGP as a form of palliation of the consequences of postoperative functional ileus (gastric distension, nausea and vomiting) for years. The probe is inserted beforehand to protect the digestive anastomosis and reduce the anastomotic dehiscence rate. It was thought that this endoluminal device could reduce the incidence of complications of the surgical wound, like eviscerations, infections and incisional hernias [16].

The use of NGP does, however, present its own morbility, which includes fever, atelectasis, pneumopathy, vomiting, gastroesophageal reflux and peptic stenosis of the oesophagus, as well as inhalation [7].

Many studies (Bauer et al.) have demonstrated that routine use of NGP is not necessary; many patients find it uncomfortable, and almost the same complications can be seen with or without its use [17].

Colvin and others compared the use and non-use of NGP during surgery and noted that there were no statistical differences, particularly in reducing the occurrence of anastomotic leakage.

Another prospective randomized study by Racette et al. in patients undergoing elective colorectal surgery found that morbidity and postoperative stay matched in both groups [18].

These studies revealed that only 7% of patients undergoing rectal surgery experienced gastric distension and vomiting, requiring the re-positioning of the NGP.

The clear conclusion to be drawn is that the use of NGP in the postoperative course of colorectal surgery must be selective and not habitual, since early feeding is tolerated well and is a benefit; furthermore, the evidence in meta-analysis and in prospective randomized studies demonstrates that the NGP:

- does not prevent postoperative ileus;
- does not prevent complications of the surgical wound (evisceration, infection, incisional hernia);
- causes nasopharyngeal complications and increases breathing difficulties caused by inhalation.

In conclusion, it may be added that the use of NGP has the logical function during a surgical operation of allowing aspiration of the air that accidentally entered the stomach at the moment of intubation, but at the same time it should be removed before the patient wakes from the anesthesia, to improve respiratory efficiency and a quick return to feeding [16].

6.8 Bladder Catheter

Urinary drainage consists in inserting a transurethral or percutaneous probe (sovrapubic catheter or epicystostomy).

In rectal surgery the bladder catheter is used: preventively to control diuresis during the surgical operation, to reduce the volume of the bladder (considering that its anatomical position hinders surgery), and for healing purposes in the event of acute urine retention (affecting 24% of men and 15% of women).

Inserting a bladder catheter creates complications like the following:

- infections of the urinary tract which range from 2 to 3 % (the commonest hospital infection) and which depend on how long the catheter remains in place, on the colonization of the collection bag, on the presence of diabetes mellitus, on the absence of antibiotic therapy, and on sex;
- formation of false tracts (primarily in male patients).

The use of a sovrapublic catheter reduces the risk of urinary infection and is more comfortable for men compared to the urinary catheter in the event of drainage lasting more than five days (long duration), even if there may be more bleeding. The risk of acute urine retention is similar for the two techniques, but the sovrapubic catheter reduces postcatheter urine disorders; in spite of this, however, it is less commonly used.

A short catheterization period, meaning 1 day, can suffice for most patients, but longer catheterization (2-3 days) is recommended in patients with low rectal cancer or previous urinary disorders [7].

Studies have demonstrated the importance of monitoring diuresis after anterior resection of the rectum in patients with epidural anesthesia. However, keeping the bladder catheter in place for more than a day seems to be counterproductive to quick mobilization [19].

6.9 Abdominal Drainage

Anastomotic leakage remains the major cause of morbidity and mortality in rectal surgery, particularly in patients with intraperitoneal anastomosis.

Studies have demonstrated that mortality from anastomotic leakage after anterior resection of the rectum stands at 12%.

The factors which make this complication more likely are : 1) neoadjuvant treatment using pelvic radiotherapy, 2) the degree of difficulty in performing the anastomosis, 3) the site of the anastomosis (the lower it is the greater the possibility of a leak), 4) total mesorectal excision, 5) the presence of intraoperative septic conditions [20].

A prospective study of 978 patients demonstrated that the appearance of an anastomotic leakage after anterior rectal resection varies from 2.9% to 12%; furthermore, it has been observed that the use of pelvic drainage, whether it be used in aspiration or in irrigation, may reduce morbidity in patients undergoing lower anterior resection of the rectum, in that the presence of this instrument allows an early removal of the material present in the abdomen (whether it be pus, hematic or enteric) [20].

On the other hand, two clinical trials have highlighted how the prophylactic use of pelvic drainage does not improve anastomotic leakage and in some cases may be damaging.

It has recently been demonstrated that no benefits derive from positioning a drainage tube because: 1) the liquid present in the abdominal cavity cannot be drained; 2) the prophylactic use of drainage after elective resection surgery neither improves the outcome nor affects the severity of the complications; 3) early diagnosis of anastomotic leakage cannot necessarily be taken for granted when drainage is present; 4) it may be painful for the patient and thus may delay discharge from hospital.

In spite of this data, highlighted in a small number of patients, there is a tendency to position a pelvic drainage tube in the perianastomotic area, particularly when the operation is particularly difficult or to prevent a pelvic hematoma; however, it merely wastes time in colon surgery.

There are different kinds of drainage: 1) drainage with irrigation-aspiration, 2) silastic drainage (silicone Penrose drainage tubes); 3) Jackson-Pratt type drainage (silicone connected to a vacuum). Suction-irrigation drainage is made up of a silicone pipe covered by a latex sheath, where the irrigation fluid (lactated Ringer's solution) is usually inserted at 60 ml per hour for 5 days after the operation, while the aspiration pressure varies from 20 to 30 cm H_2O [21].

6.10 Quick Mobilization

It has been demonstrated that an extended stay in bed increases insulin resistance, reduces strength and muscle tone, reduces lung function as a consequence oxygenation of the tissues, and in addition increases the risk of thromboembolism.

Good pain control is the key to rapid mobilization, because it is the presence of pain that often slows out-of-bed time; it follows that a pre-established assistance plan may be useful for this purpose. The presence of abdominal drainage or a urinary catheter may also slow down mobilization, so that it is important that these instruments are removed as early as possible.

Early mobilization may be useful for inducing intestinal activity and thus reducing postoperative ileus; as a consequence there is earlier recovery of peristalsis and along with it defecation.

In patients undergoing surgical operations of elective anterior resection of the rectum the objective is therefore to get them out of bed for 2 hours on the day of the operation itself and for 6 hours on the subsequent days until they are discharged [3].

This regime helps the patient to improve not only physically but also psychologically, with a consequent reduction of hospitalization.

6.11 Conclusions

The reduction of postoperative mortality and morbidity in operations of anterior resection of the rectum is linked to surgical and anesthetic techniques, as well as to an improvement in perioperative management, which has changed radically in the last few years.

A cornerstone element is the correct preparation of the intestine before surgery, which shows a tendency to be standardized in less drastic forms; feeding both before and after the operation is also of crucial importance.

Anesthesia plays an important role not only during induction, but also in postoperative analgesic treatment, which is often essential for a quick recovery of the patient and with it short hospitalization.

Early removal of the various instruments (nasogastric tube, bladder catheter, abdominal drainage) used during the hospital stay is aimed at reducing the onset of complications, aiding a quick recovery and improving the outcome.

References

1. Napolitano LM (2005) Standardization of perioperative management: clinical pathways. Surg Clin North Am 85:1321-1327
2. Kehlet H, Dahl JB (2003) Anastesia, surgery, and challenges in postoperative recovery. Lancet 6:1921-1928
3. Lassen K, Soop M, Nygren J et al (2009) Consensus Review of optimal perioperative care in colorectal surgery: Enhanced Recovery After Surgery (ERAS) Group recommendations. Arch Surg 144:961-969
4. Roig JV, Gracia-Fadrique A, Redondo C et al (2008) Perioperative care in colorectal surgery: current practice patterns and opinions. Colorectal Dis 11: 976-983
5. Polle SW, Wind J, Fuhring JW et al (2007) Implementation of a fast-track perioperative care program: what are the difficulties? Dig Surg 24:441-449
6. Jung B, Lannerstad O, Påhlman L et al (2007) Preoperative mechanical preparation of colon: the patient's experience. BMC Surgery 7:1-5
7. Mariette C, Slim K (2007) Trattamento perioperatorio in chirurgia digestiva. EMC, Tecniche Chirurgiche, pp 40-45
8. Bretagnol F, Panis Y, Rullier E et al (2010) Rectal cancer surgery with or without bowel preparation: The French GRECCAR III multicenter single-blinded randomized trial. Ann Surg 252:863-868
9. Guenaga KF, Matos D, Wille-Jørgensen P (2011) Mechanical bowel preparation for elective colorectal surgery. Cochrane Database Syst Rev. Issue 9
10. Scabini S, Rimini E, Romairone E et al (2010) Colon and rectal surgery for cancer without mechanical bowel preparation: one-center randomized prospective trial. World J Surg Oncol 8:35-39
11. Craig DG, Bates CM, Davidson JS et al (2011) Staggered overdose pattern and delay to hospital presentation are associated with adverse outcomes following paracetamol-induced hepatotoxicity. Br J Clin Pharmacol 73:285-294
12. Berggvist D, Agnelli G, Cohen AT et al (2002) Duration of prophylaxis against venous thromboembolism with enoxaparin after surgery for cancer. N Engl J Med 346:975-979
13. Businger A, Grunder G, Guenin MO et al (2011) Mechanical bowel preparation and antimicrobial prophylaxis in elective colorectal surgery in Switzerland-a survey. Langenbecks Arch Surg 396:107-113
14. Zelenitsky SA, Ariano RE, Harding GK, Silverman RE (2002) Antibiotic Pharmacodynamics in Surgical Prophylaxis: an Association between Intraoperative Antibiotic Concentrations and Efficacy. Antimicrob Agents Chemother 46:3026-3030
15. Chen Y, Liu BL, Shang B, Chen AS et al (2011) Nutrition support in surgical patients with colorectal cancer. World J Gastroenterol 17:1779-1786
16. Villalba Ferrer F, Bruna Esteban M, García Coret MJ et al (2007) Evidence of early oral feeding in colorectal surgery. Rev Esp Enfer Dig 99:709-713

17. Bauer JJ, Gelernt IM, Salky BA et al (1985) Is a routine postoperative nasogastric decompression really necessary? Ann Surg 201:233-236
18. Racette DL, Chang FC, Trekell ME, Farha GJ (1987) Is Nasogastric intubation necessary in colon operations? Am J Surg 154:640-642
19. O'Kelly TJ, Mathew A, Ross S, Munro A (1995) Optimum method for urinary drainage in major abdominal surgery: a prospective randomized trial of sovrapubic vs urethral catheterization. Br J Surg 82:1367-1368
20. Alves A, Panis Y, Trancart D et al (2002) Factors Associated with Clinically Significant Anastomotic Leakage after Large Bowel Resection: Multivariate Analysis of 707 Patients. World J Surg 26:499-502
21. Yeh CY, Changchien CR, Wang JY et al (2005) Pelvic Drainage and Other Risk Factors for Leakage After Elective Anterior Resection in Rectal Cancer Patient. Ann Surg 241:9-13

Surgical Technique 7

Paola Tarchi, Davide Cosola and Nicolò de Manzini

7.1 Introduction

In this chapter we analyze the surgical technique of rectal resections, focusing on describing the laparoscopic approach and our usual technique.

The laparoscopic surgical set includes the usual instruments, which means atraumatic grasping forceps, dissector, clip applier, and a suction-irrigation system. Furthermore each surgeon should use the dissection-coagulation system that he or she is most familiar with (bipolar, ultrasounds, radiofrequency), as there is no particular standard set of instruments. Linear, angular or circular staplers for transanal mechanical anastomosis can also be chosen.

7.2 Position of the Patient and the Surgical Team

The position of the patient and the surgical team in the operating room are now standardized. Our practice is to use a non-slip gel mattress on the operating table, avoiding any restraints that may lead to a risk of lesions to the brachial plexus. The patient is placed supine in a gynecological position using Allen stirrups as a support for the lower limbs, which are divaricated and raised, especially during the perineal phase. The left arm is placed at right angles to allow positioning of and access to an A-V line and the pulse oximeter. A vesical catheter is always inserted, and if there are problems of catheterization due to prostate disease, it is advisable to wait and position an epicys-

P. Tarchi (✉)
Department of Medicine, Surgery and Health Sciences, General Surgery Unit,
Cattinara University Hospital,
Trieste, Italy
e-mail: paolatarchi@hotmail.com

N. de Manzini (ed.), *Rectal Cancer*,
Updates in Surgery
DOI: 10.1007/978-88-470-2670-4_7, © Springer-Verlag Italia 2013

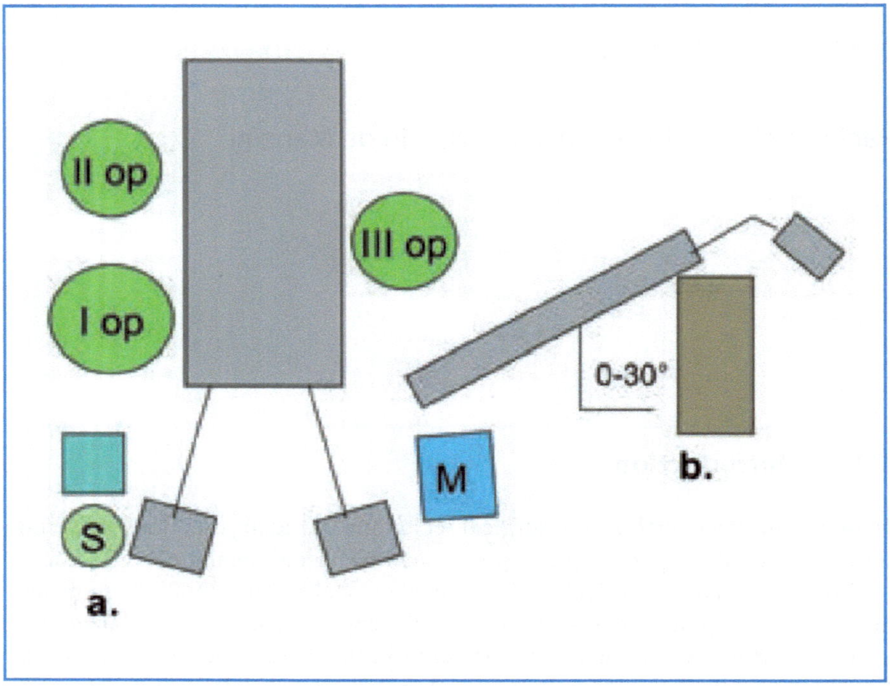

Fig. 7.1 Position of the operating table and surgical team. The patient is placed in a flat supine position with the lower extremities in Dan Allen stirrups, with open legs, and only minimally elevated above the abdomen. Both the surgeon and the camera holder stand on the patient's right side, a third optional operator between the legs. The main monitor is located in front of the surgeon, on the left side of the patient

tostomy under visual control, once the operation has started. A naso-gastric tube is not positioned routinely, but may be specifically requested by the surgeon if gastric distension is found on exploring the abdomen.

The surgeon and the cameraman stand on the right side of the patient, the third assistant between the patient's legs and the scrub nurse to the right of the surgeon (Fig. 7.1). The laparoscopic column is positioned on the left side and the high definition monitor at the patient's feet at the height of the patient's left flank, opposite the surgeon. A second monitor may be useful. During the first phase of the operation, the vascular phase, the operating table remains horizontal but is rotated towards the right, whereas during the pelvic phase the right rotation is maintained but a Trendelenburg position of at least 30° is required.

The standard positioning of the 5 trocars used for anterior resection is illustrated in Figure 7.2. The 10 mm optic trocar is introduced 4 cm above the umbilicus in a median position using an open technique. Pneumoperitoneum is induced at 14 mmHg and then two 5 mm trocars are positioned under visual

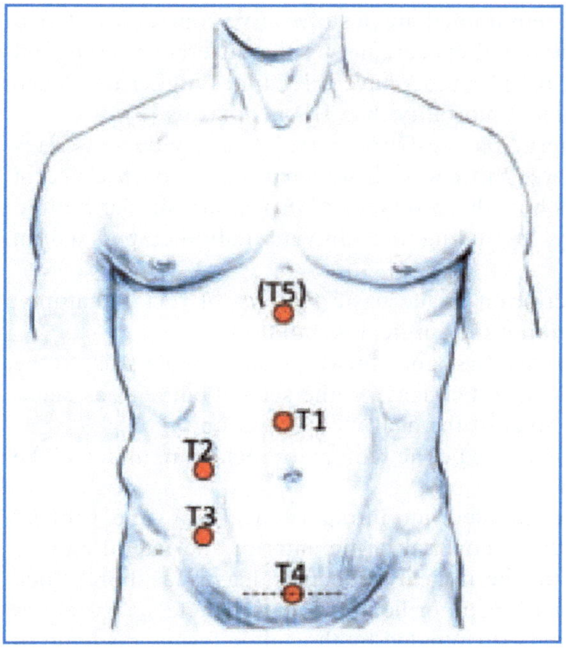

Fig. 7.2 Trocar positions for laparoscopic Total Mesorectal Excision of rectal cancer.
The position of the camera trocar is 4 cm above the umbilicus, two 5-mm trocars are located below the xiphoid and in the right upper quadrant, a 12-mm port is placed in the right lower quadrant and the 12-mm suprapubic trocar is placed where the Pfannenstiel incision will be made

control, respectively in the epigastric region and in the right hypochondrium along the emiclavear line. A 12 mm trocar is then inserted 2 cm above and medially to the anterior superior iliac spine, and a 12 mm port in the sovrapubic region. At this point a minilaparotomy incision is made to extract the surgical specimen. However, there are many variants of the position of the trocars as well as of the choice of minilaparotomy. These variants do not differ significantly from what we have described above [1].

As during any laparoscopic procedure, there must always be the possibility of conversion at any time during the operation. An instrument table with the basic instruments needed for a laparotomy should therefore be kept ready.

7.3 Surgical Anatomy

The treatment of rectal cancer has undergone a significant evolution over the last ten years, with progressive improvements in terms of surgical technique, technology and oncological results.

Two different situations must be distinguished in rectal cancer: that of neoplasms situated in the high rectum (HR), roughly located above the Douglas pouch, conventionally between 10 and 15 cm from the anal margin; and that of middle and low rectal cancers, located below 10 cm from the anal verge, which corresponds to the extraperitoneal rectum. This division appears to be fully justified both by the different immediate postoperative course, with twice as many complications for low rectal cancer, and by the different oncological results at 5 years: in fact, low rectal tumors have a 1.9 times higher incidence of local relapse and cancer-related mortality than HR neoplasms [2].

A comparison of the long-term disease-free survival data also demonstrates how HR cancer does not differ significantly from what has been observed in sigmoid cancer [3], and shows how the two types of cancer are similar both in terms of therapeutic strategy, excluding neoadjuvant radiotherapy, and in terms of oncological results.

There follows a brief description of the basic features of rectal anatomy, which will be helpful in describing the surgical techniques.

The rectum has two curves: the first goes forwards and downwards, to the levator complex, following the sacral concavity; the second curve goes backwards and downwards, to the level of the anal-rectal junction.

The rectum can be divided into the pelvic rectum, or rectal ampulla, and the perineal rectum, or anal canal.

The pelvic rectum is further divided into intraperitoneal and subperitoneal portions. In the first, the rectum is covered in the anterior and lateral part by the peritoneum; posteriorly the peritoneal reflection leaves a short, thick mesorectum containing the upper rectal or hemorrhoidal pedicle.

The extra-peritoneal rectum is surrounded by the pelvic fascia, made up of two membranes: the visceral membrane, or mesorectal fascia, which surrounds the rectum, and the parietal sheet of the pelvic fascia. In males, from the anterior face of the rectum the peritoneum reflects onto the posterior surface of the seminal vesicles, of the vas deferens and of the bladder, forming the Douglas rectovesical pouch and the rectoprostatic Denonvilliers' fascia; in females, it reflects onto the posterior surface of the vagina and of the uterus, creating the rectovaginal septum. The end of the rectovaginal septum is positioned lower than the rectovesical pouch: the distance between the blind end and the anus is 5.5 cm in women and 7.5 cm in men. Posteriorly, the rectum comes into relation with the anterior face of the sacrum, covered by the parietal membrane (also known as the presacral fascia or Waldeyer's fascia) and by its reinforcement called the rectosacral ligament. This fascia provides posterior support to the rectum and contributes to maintaining its sacrococcygeal angle. Laterally the peritoneal reflection creates pararectal recesses. The lateral pararectal space contains the ureters, the hypogastric vessels and their branches, as well as the nerve structures related to the sacro-rectal-genito-pubic ligaments. From here the lateral ligaments become detached in a frontal plane, representing a means of fixing the mesorectum to the lateral walls of the pelvis; the lateral ligaments are not actually an anatomic entity but "structures" created by the tension connected to the upward traction on the rectum during surgical dissection. The median rectal artery runs inside the lateral ligaments in less than a third of cases, and is more often present only on one side, whereas the presence of rectal nerve branches coming from the lateral pelvic plexus is much more constant.

The mesorectum, described for the first time by Heald [4] in 1982, is made up of cellular fatty tissue, which surrounds the subperitoneal rectum, more abundantly on the posterior-lateral sides and thinner along the anterior face. It is surrounded by a thin, connective, dense lamina, called Jonnesco's fibrous sheath of the rectum or Waldeyer's fascia (mesorectal fascia), a visceral reflection on the pelvic fascia. This fascia gets progressively thinner towards the most distal portion of the viscera in proximity to the levator muscles, leaving a segment of 2 cm completely without mesorectum.

The mesorectum contains the branches of vessel and nerve divisions destined to the rectum and the perirectal lymph nodes, of fundamental importance in the regional spread of neoplasms of the middle and lower rectum.

There is an avascular dissection space (Heald's *holy plane*) between the parietal and visceral sheets of the pelvic fascia in the connective cellular fatty tissue of the presacral space, which should be followed during surgical resection, respecting the integrity of the mesorectal fascia and guaranteeing a complete exeresis of the mesorectum.

The perineal rectum or anal canal, about 4 cm long, passes through the pelvic diaphragm, made up of the puborectal sling of the levator muscle of the anus, whose fibers reach those of the deep part of the external sphincter. At this level there is no spontaneously cleavable perirectal plane. In men the anal canal relates anteriorly to the tendinous centre of the perineum, the urogenital diaphragm which contains the membranous portion of the urethra; in women it relates to the perineal middle and posterior vaginal wall. Laterally the anal canal is in relation to the ischioanal fossa. The sphincteric apparatus is made up of two rings of muscle: the internal and the external sphincters, separated by an intermediate layer of vertical fibers. The internal sphincter is made up of smooth fibers and forms a muscular sleeve, which surrounds the upper three quarters of the anal canal for about 3 cm and guarantees involuntary continence with its tone. The external sphincter is made up of striated muscle fibers and surrounds the internal sphincter, ensuring voluntary continence. It is made up of three bundles: the deep one surrounds the upper portion of the anal canal; the upper fibers continue with the puborectal fascia of the levator muscle of the anus, from which it cannot be distinguished; finally, its surface bundle has an elliptic form and surrounds the lower half of the internal sphincter up to the anocutaneous line. The complex longitudinal layer is made up of smooth fibers coming from the longitudinal muscle layer of the rectum, of striated fibers coming from the levator of the anus and other tendinous fibers deriving from the pelvic aponeurosis. This muscle-tendon structure extends downwards into the intersphincteric space. The lower portion of the internal sphincter is surrounded by these fibers, which form the Parks ligament.

The arterial supply of the rectum derives from the superior rectal artery, the terminal branch of the lower mesenteric artery and of the middle and lower rectal arteries. The upper rectal artery, after entering the mesorectum at the level of the third sacral vertebra, divides into two branches, right and left, and is the most important source of blood supply, vascularizing all the pelvic rectum and the mucosa of the anal canal. The middle rectal artery comes from the hypogastric artery and moves transversely to the levator muscle below the lateral ligament, vascularising the extraperitoneal portion of the rectum. As already seen, its presence is not constant, 22% monolateral, and of modest calibre. The lower rectal artery comes from the pudendal artery, goes towards the ischiorectal fossa and vascularises the internal and external anal sphincter, the levator muscle of the anus and the submucosa of the anal canal. Finally, the sacral artery comes from the aortic bifurcation, and goes down along the median line in front of the sacral but behind the presacral fascia.

Venous blood is conveyed to the mesenteric-portal system mainly through the IMV, but is also, to a lesser extent, a tributary of the caval system through the hypogastric veins. In the posterior mobilization of the rectum, great care must be taken to avoid lesion (disinsertion) to the presacral venous plexus tributary of the inferior caval system, connected by means of the basivertebral veins with the internal vertebral venous plexus.

Lymphatic drainage of the rectum moves cranially, starting parallel to the arterial vessels.

The lymphatic vessels are organized in an intramural (submucous, intermuscular and mesorectal) and an extramural plexus. The upper portion of the extramural plexus drains the intraperitoneal rectum and only partially the extraperitoneal rectum, following the course of the superior rectal artery towards the inferior mesenteric lymph nodes (Bacon axilla, the origin of the IMA), and from here towards the preaortic nodes. The lymphatic vessels of the middle and low rectum and the anal canal drain laterally towards the perineal structures through the sphincters and the levator muscles, but also upwards outside the mesorectal fascia and only rarely towards the internal iliac vessels. The lower pedicle drains the pelvic distal rectum and the anal canal above the pectinate line and, following the inferior rectal vessels, reaches the obturator iliac lymph nodes, while below the pectinate line the lymph is conveyed in the direction of the superficial inguinal nodes.

The innervation of the rectum is made up of a sympathetic component coming from the roots of L1, L2 and L3, which constitutes the pre-aortic or intermesenteric plexus, located in front of the aorta, which connects to the superior hypogastric plexus: the left one comes extremely close to the inferior mesenteric vessels, whereas the right one is positioned further behind the level of the aorto-caval corner. The presacral plexus divides immediately under the promontory of the sacrum into two pelvic or hypogastic nerves, which run parallel and medially to the ureters. These nerves come into contact with the postero-superior surface of the mesorectum, outside the peri-rectal fascia, ending in the inferior or pelvic hypogastric plexus. The lowest portion of this plexus approaches the mesorectum and is located anterior and inferior to the lateral ligament of the rectum, which contains the rectal branches. Male ejaculation and female vaginal lubrication depend on the pelvic plexus.

The parasympathetic roots originating from S2, S3 and S4 are, however, responsible for erection. They run across the front face of the pyramidal muscles under the pelvic aponeurosis, and can be highlighted in the presacral space by moving the mesorectum forwards. The erector nerves come from the sacral parasympathetic system, joining the fibers of the sympathetic system at the lateral pelvic plexus, and from here send terminations to the pelvic organs.

7.4 An Important Issue: Margins

The anatomopathological status of resection margins is with no doubt one of the most important prognostic factors in rectal neoplasm surgery .

In the 1960s Grinnell found an extended distal intramural spread in 12% of rectal and recto-sigmoid cancers, sometimes up to 4 cm from the lower margin of the neoplasia; he recommended extending the resection to 5 cm below the inferior macroscopic margin [2]. This recommendation became a rule, to the extent that 70% of rectal cancers were treated with abdominoperineal amputation (APR), which at the time represented the gold standard for middle and low rectal tumors.

The revision of the 5 cm rule and the introduction of staplers, which made low or ultra-low colorectal anastomosis almost always technically possible, meant that this "sphincter saving" surgery could be extended.

The finding of a submucous intramural distal diffusion in up to 40% of cases of rectal carcinoma, but with an extension greater than 1 cm only in 4-6% of cases, led to a redefinition of a distal resection margin of only 2 cm as more oncologically correct. Thus APR was indicated only for carcinomas less than 5 cm from the anal verge or less than 2 cm from the anal ring.

In 1995 Scott pointed out the presence of neoplastic deposits in the mesorectum, discontinuous with respect to rectal carcinoma, up to 5 cm below the neoplasia [2]; accordingly, a new resection margin was defined, the "distal margin of the mesorectum", whose optimal extension meant a systematic total excision of the mesorectum (TME) in low rectum cancer (Fig. 7.3). The widespread adoption of TME, proposed by Heald in 1982 [4], led to the identification of a third resection margin, the "circumferential margin" (CRM), determined by the millimetric distance between the mesorectal fascia and the most lateral margin of the tumor or any metastatic lymphadenopathy (Fig. 7.4). This has played a fundamental prognostic role in terms of local recurrence (from 2% to 11% at 5 years in the event of positivity), as well as being a factor of primary choice, as regards both the decision to use neoadjuvant radiochemiotherapy and its duration. Thus today a correct histological study of the operative specimen must also be performed on transversal sections, to analyze the radial clearance and not to miss an infiltration of the circumferential section which has the same negative prognostic value as an infiltrated distal section.

The multimodal treatment of locally advanced low rectum carcinoma improved the local control of the disease and allowed a further increase in sphincter-saving procedures: today, by associating neoadjuvant radiochemiotherapy (RCT) to TME, sphincter conservation can be achieved in 70% of

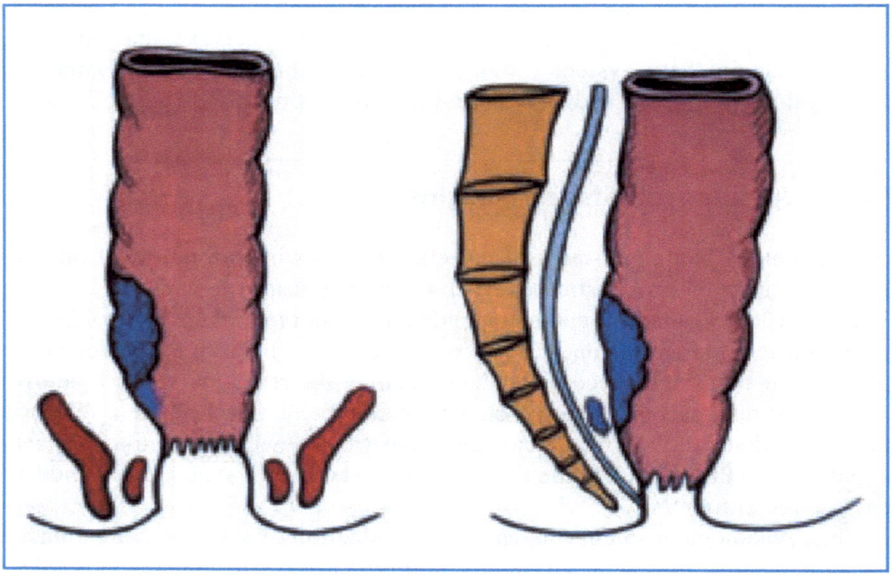

Fig. 7.3 Distal intramural margin and mesorectal distal spread

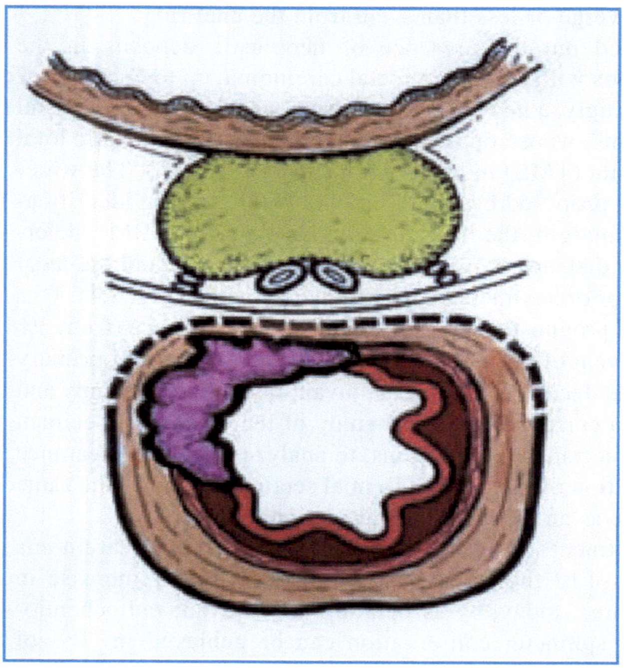

Fig. 7.4 Mesorectal fascia in black, allowing the measurement of distance from lateral tumor spread

cases of low rectal carcinomas [5]. In these cases the distal resection margin can be reduced to 1 cm [6], and still be considered as oncologically safe, thus allowing procedures like partial or total intersphincteric resection (as proposed by Rullier), even for carcinomas located less than 4.5 cm from the anal margin or with the lower margin less than 2 cm from the dentate line [7].

The tumor shrinkage effect, the result of the response of the neoplasia to neoadjuvant treatment, is at the basis of this further lowering of the distal resection margin [8], and makes it necessary to reconsider the choice of the most appropriate surgery 4-6 weeks from the end of RCT, when tumor regression seems more important, although at that date it is disputable.

The latest data from the Dutch TME Trial show how neoadjuvant RCT can lead to a reduction of local relapses, even with a distal margin just above 5 mm [3, 9-12].

7.5 Vascular Phase

During this phase the operating table is rotated to the right side of the patient, to make the Treitz ligament easier to see. The forceps inserted into the epigastric trocar lifts the lower face of the transverse mesocolon, while the hypogastric forceps grasps the vascular pedicle, which can be viewed by lifting the sigma, straining the lower mesenteric vein . This type of exposure allows a clear, stable vision of the vascular elements, and in our opinion is the basic position for those starting this kind of surgery.

The first jejunal portion needs to be lifted from the retroperitoneum in order to correctly expose the aortic plane and the emergence of the IMV.

An incision of the peritoneum is then made below the IMV, and Toldt's fascia is lifted up to the lower margin of the pancreas (cranially) and up to the lateral descending colon; in this phase the left ureter, the gonadic vessels and the lower edge of the tail of the pancreas can be recognized.

The IMV is then bound and cut below the pancreas, while the artery is prepared subadventitially and may be cut either at its origin (high tie) or after the emergence of the left colic artery (low tie); ever since Miles and Moynihan respectively proposed the techniques of low and high tie of the IMA, there has been significant debate regarding which of the two techniques is preferable.

No randomized controlled study has tried to clear up the dilemma, but even the several non-randomized or retrospective studies analyzed in two recent reviews [13, 14] do not demonstrate a clear advantage of either technique in terms of global and disease-free survival or complications (anastomotic leaks or stenosis, sexual or urinary dysfunctions).

The supporters of the "low tie" technique highlight the uselessness of a more invasive and more destructive operation without any oncologic benefit [15], especially in the less advanced stages, exposing the patient to greater risk of hypoperfusion to the proximal colic stump [16] and possible damage to the structures of the autonomous nervous systems [13].

On the other hand, if the high tie is performed at the origin of the IMA, it should be safer for the hypogastric plexus, which never meets the arterial axis [17] at this level, and pose a smaller risk of tension to the anastomosis caused by the left colic artery (LCA)/IMA axis, as well as permitting a better lymphadenectomy [7]. Although it has been demonstrated that harvesting 12 nodes is sufficient to guarantee the correct oncological radicality and disease-free survival [14, 18], a number of patients could benefit from lymphadenectomy up to the origin of the IMA, in terms of radicality and complete staging [14].

However, it is well known that the localization of the lymph-nodes at the origin of the IMA is related, in most cases, to systemic dissemination of the disease (which would explain why the high tie does not give any statistically significant survival advantage) [19, 20].

Furthermore, awareness of the possible pathological effects of these lymph node stations does not currently involve the application of different or additional therapeutic strategies but at the most a more careful follow-up [19].

Our experience leads us to prefer a high-tie approach, not only for the undoubted advantages that this provides in laparoscopy (absence of tension to the anastomosis, easier approach to posterior dissection), but also so that even the very small percentage of patients with tumoral localization at the apical stations without systemic dissemination either present or latent can benefit from a radical oncological operation.

Furthermore, in our experience (which is supported by literature citations) patients are not exposed to a greater risk of anastomotic complications or autonomic nerve plexus lesions.

After the vascular phase, an incision is performed in the left parieto-colic gutter with splenic flexure mobilization; a gauze above Gerota's fascia during dissection of Toldt's fascia may help to protect the ureters and the gonadic vessels from mechanical or thermal injury, as well as highlighting the right cleavage plane during dissection of the paracolic gutter. The mobilization of the distal third of the transverse colon is advisable in any case, but especially in laparoscopy, where the tension of the lowered colon can only be assessed visually. This manoeuvre can be performed either cranially or caudally; sometimes it is necessary to open the gastrocolic ligament. Basically, all the different possibilities must be known to adapt the procedure to each individual case.

It should be pointed out that in laparotomy, and for some authors in laparoscopy, a lateromedial approach is normally preferred, starting from an incision along Monk's line and continuing medially until the mesenteric vessels are reached.

7.6 Pelvic Phase

During this phase the operating table is placed in the Trendelenburg position with an inclination close to 30°.

The pelvic phase starts with an incision of the peritoneum laterally to the rectum and anteriorly to the right iliac vessels and then continues anteriorly to the anterior wall of the rectouterine pouch, about 2 cm above its reflection (this allows a solid point of traction for dissecting the mesorectal fascia from the posterior wall of the vagina or from the vesico-prostatic plane). Posteriorly the mesorectal fascia is dissected from Waldeyer's presacral fascia, helped by the traction on the inferior mesenteric artery stump, being careful to preserve the nerve structures, which run anterior to the promontory.

The rectosacral fascia has significant surgical importance: when not respected, its section can lead to perforation of the rectum or hemorrhage of the presacral venous plexus, as can a dissection carried out too close to the visceral or sacral wall. Secondly, the complete mobilization of the mesorectum is not possible without the transversal division of the rectosacral fascia, reaching in this way the levator muscle plane.

Respecting the mesorectal fascia and Heald's plan is no longer a matter of debate in terms of oncological safety, survival and relapse rates [4, 21].

Considering the role of the margins and technical progress in reconstruction, the Miles' abdominoperineal amputation is today restricted to cases of infiltration of the external sphincter and/or levator muscle or to patients affected by incontinence.

7.7 PME and TME

Since, as we said before, the mesorectum must be cut at least 5 cm distally to the tumor, it is clear that partial mesorectal excision (PME) is only applicable to high rectal tumors; in all other cases a total mesorectal excision (TME) must be performed. In both cases the technique is almost the same, differing as regards the level of depth. After the incision of the peritoneum as described above, we deepen the distal dissection respecting the integrity of the mesorectal fascia, progressively exposed by the traction and countertraction movements of the rectum and of the extraperitoneal fibroadipose tissue; anteriorly the peritoneal reflection portion should be used as a solid traction point (Figs. 7.5, 7.6). In this phase it is essential never to grasp the rectum at the level of the neoplasia, respecting the no-touch technique, but above all to expose the surgical field. In that way the mesorectal fascia remains uninterrupted, guaranteeing the oncological value of the dissection (Fig. 7.7).

The tying of the superior and middle rectal vessels is also performed during mesorectal excision; clips, slow resorption thread, ultrasound scalpels or bipolar forceps may be used.

Once a suitable level of depth has been reached, or, in the case of TME, the level of the pelvic floor, the section is continued in the direction of the rectal wall; at this point the distal section can be performed using a mechanical linear stapler (Fig. 7.8). This manoeuvre may be difficult in the event of bulky tumors in narrow pelvis. In these cases there may be a temptation to section the rectum even lower, transanally, thus lowering the section line beyond the

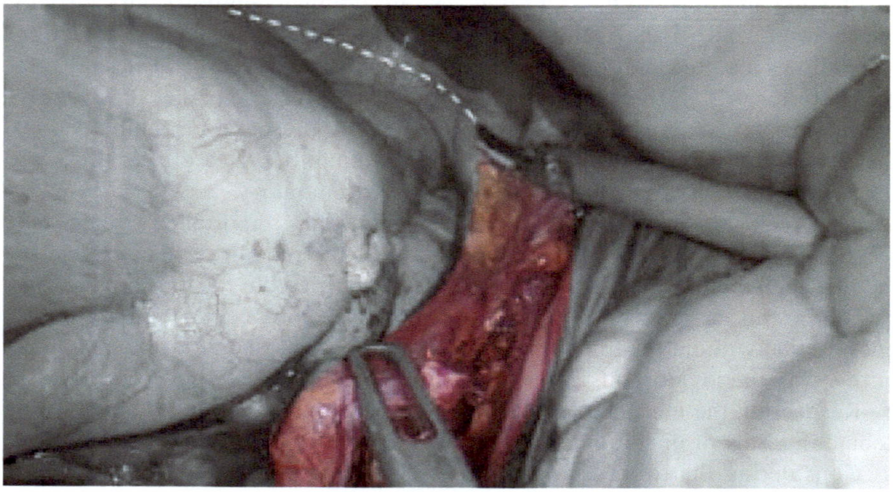

Fig. 7.5 Anterior opening of the peritoneum, taking care to stay on the vesical/vaginal side, in order to have a solid point of traction and to respect the integrity of the anterior part of mesorectal fascia

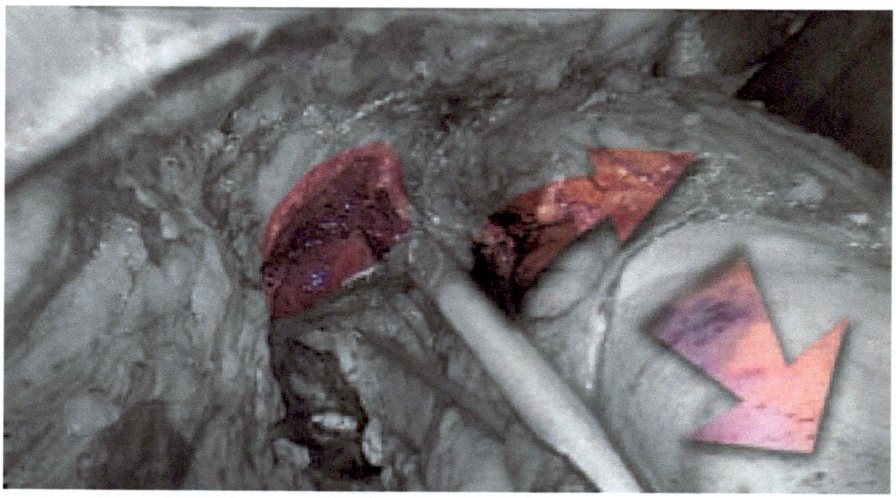

Fig. 7.6 The double movement of traction (*straight arrow*) by a proximal grasper, and countertraction (*curved arrow*) allows widening of the lateral part of the mesorectum, which is easily dissected

formal oncological limit and increasing the risk of sequelae: this grey zone, situated in the submesorectal rectum, should, however, be preserved if possible. However, there are significant technical possibilities, like inserting the linear stapler in the hypogastric trocar [22] or using open-surgery angled or

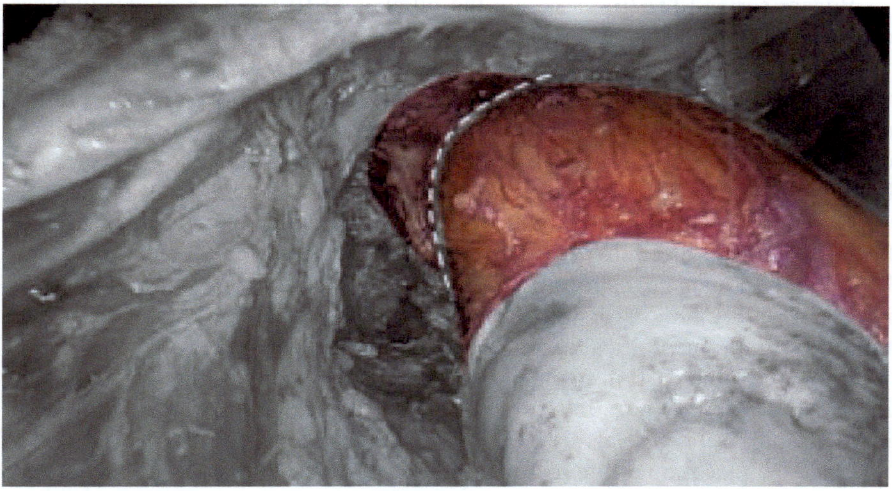

Fig. 7.7 Once mesorectal dissection is complete, the submesorectal part of the rectum becomes visible (after dashed line)

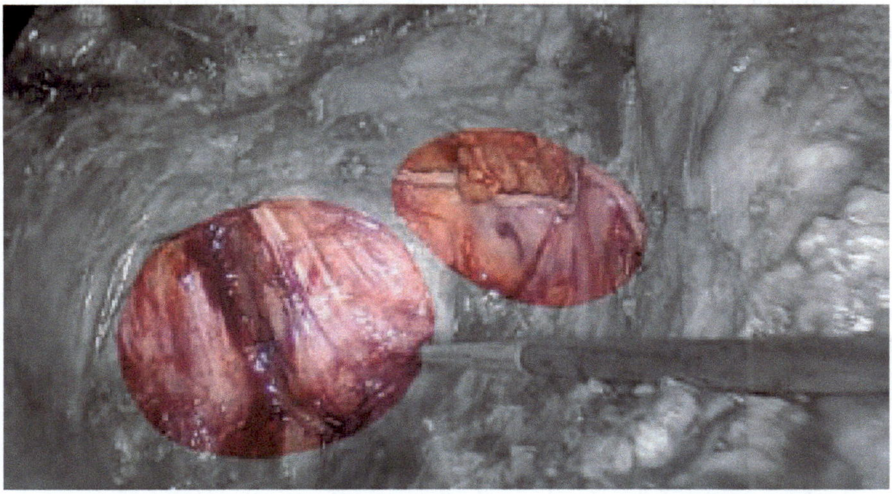

Fig. 7.8 Final view after TME resection: the linear stapled line is visible and the left levator muscle is completely visible, confirming complete TME

curved staplers after a Pfannenstiel minilaparotomy [23, 24]. More recently the use of the transanal endoscopic technique (the same as that used for TEM) has been proposed, even though there is not yet sufficient evidence in literature for its use in this approach [25].

Recent series [22, 26] associate the number of firings to a higher number of anastomotic dehiscences.

In particular two studies recently demonstrated a reduction of the incidence from 15% to 3% (p=0.02) [22] if less than three firings are used. This result is also confirmed in the work of Kim et al. [26] in which, furthermore, the incidence drops to 1.1% if a single firing is used (8.9% in the event of two firings), but with a borderline statistical significance (p=0.08).

Our experience suggests that the use of a 45 mm stapler is advisable, because this very often involves two firings. In contrast, the 60 mm stapler can be difficult to manage, especially in a narrow pelvis, in overweight patients or in case of bulky tumors: its poor handling exposes to the risk of oblique sections with both oncological and vascular consequences.

This is not the case in open surgery, where the use of a single 60 mm firing is almost always possible, as well as the use of the above-mentioned dedicated staplers.

Once the resection of the rectum has been performed, the surgical specimen is removed via a protected minilaparotomy. It is then possible to proceed to the proximal section of the colon, and choose the reconstruction method.

Once the pneumoperitoneum has been reintroduced, intestinal continuity is re-established by means of the transanal mechanical circular stapler.

Again, the choice of the calibre must be specific for the patient, considering that a firing diameter between 25 and 29 mm is responsible for a greater number of stenoses, whereas a stapler diameter between 31 and 33 causes a greater number of anastomotic leaks, probably due to the greater distension of the distal stump [22].

7.8 Intersphincteric Resection

This operation, devised by Rullier [7], is indicated in tumors of the ultra-low rectum (surgical anal canal), which exceed the muscolaris mucosae and involve the muscular layer, which thickens at this level to form the internal sphincter, sparing the striated muscle (external sphincter and anus levator muscle).

This type of resection follows that of TME as regards the pelvic phase (described above), but also envisages a perineal phase divided into two stages:

- Circular dissection: the anal canal mucosa is cut circularly 1-2 cm below the lower pole of the neoplasia (in the case of patients eligible for neoadjuvant therapy, this level should be determined before beginning the therapy); the incision must include the whole thickness of the internal sphincter, and the dissection plane between the internal and external sphincters should be recognized first posterolaterally (where it is more evident) and then anteriorly. At this point the rectum is closed transanally;
- Longitudinal dissection: this proceeds cranially along the avascular plan between the two sphincters until it reaches the level of the postero-lateral pelvic floor at the level of the superior pole of the external sphincter ante-

riorly; at this point, following the superior fascia of the pelvic floor and Waldeyer's presacral fascia, it reaches the dissection limit obtained during the abdominal phase.

During this operation the creation of a neoampulla is always recommended, using one of the techniques described in the 9th chapter, while the extraction of the surgical specimen is carried out transanally. This manoeuvre is safe when the tumor is not locally advanced (thus in all patients eligible for intersphincteric resection), while if the tumor is greater than or equal to T3, it is as yet not clear whether the risk of neoplastic dissemination increases during the passage through the pelvic diaphragm.

7.9 Abdomino-perineal Amputation

This surgical technique, introduced by Miles more than a hundred years ago, involves removing the whole rectum, the anus and the sphincteric apparatus. As mentioned, this operation is currently recommended in ultra-low rectal cancer ineligible for trans-sphincteric resection, either because it involves the external sphincter even after neoadjuvant therapy, or due to a pre-existing patient's incontinence. The operating technique consists in an abdominal phase very similar to anterior resection with TME, and a perineal phase. The latter, in the classic technique, is performed with the patient in the lithotomy position, and starts with a rhombus- or cup-shaped incision circumscribing the anus and without involving the urethral bulb in males. This is continued into the ischiorectal fossa up to the levator plane; this muscle is sectioned just outside the striated sphincter, reaching the abdominal dissection limit. In this way the surgical specimen takes on a characteristic "egg-timer" shape due to the narrowing of the visceral passage through the pelvic floor.

Despite the TME, local relapse did not fall significantly with APR, remaining around 25-30% [27], associated to a high percentage of positivity of the CRM. This is more likely due to the changed indications, which are now more selective, involving only tumors located in close proximity to the sphincter, just where the specimen narrows. In the past, APR was also performed for higher tumors, with no or low risk of sphincter involvement.

This has led to a more extensive operation called "cylindrical or extralevator abdominoperineal amputation" [28], which has the specific purpose of increasing the amplitude of the CRM at the levator ani muscle. During the perineal phase of this operation, the patient should be put in a prone position and the incision, larger posterolaterally, may also include the coccyx posteriorly, which will be disarticulated; anteriorly it follows the same plane as the classic technique, as it must preserve the urethra in males and the posterior vaginal wall in females (unless the removal of these structures is recommended for oncological radicality).

The dissection proceeds as far as the muscular plane, which is cut very close to the obturator muscle [29].

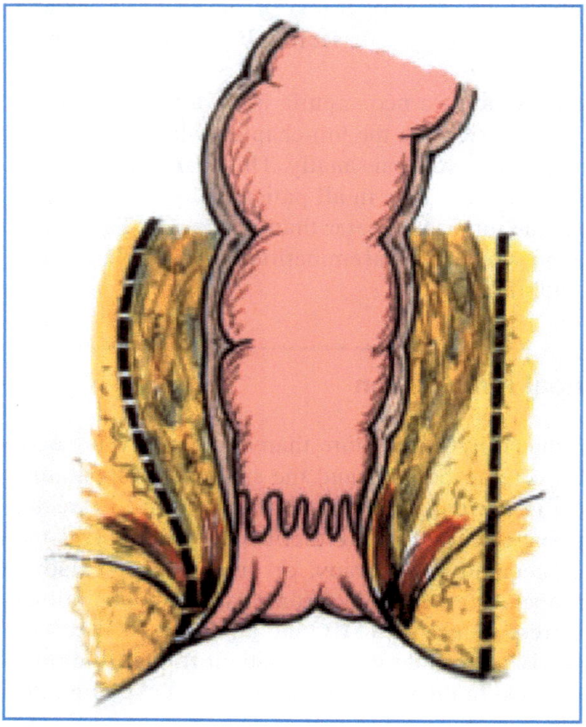

Fig. 7.9 The two different dissection planes in standard (left dashed line) and extended extralevator (*right dashed line*) abdominoperineal resection

This technique, which results in a surgical specimen of a cylindrical shape, has demonstrated a lower incidence of local relapses and a better disease-free and overall survival rate [27, 30]; however, it often requires gluteal flaps or biological meshes for the reconstruction of the perineal region, steps which complicate the procedure and postoperative morbidity [28, 29] (Fig. 7.9).

If we look at the results in terms of survival, the percentage of positive CRM (dropping from 40% to 15 %) and of intraoperatory visceral perforation (from 23% to 4%), we believe that a cylindrical amputation should be considered the surgical standard [27], in spite of the possible increase in morbidity. However, the amplitude of the surgical specimen and the structures involved may be assessed case by case on the basis of the oncological stage (the approach will be different if striated muscles are involved or if a patient with a slightly higher tumor is incontinent) and of the clinical condition of the patient.

7.10 TEM

Progressively earlier diagnosis and neoadjuvant therapy have increased the number of small rectal carcinomas that surgeons have had to deal with over the years. Transanal resection is gradually being replaced by Transanal Endoscopic Microsurgery (TEM), introduced by Buess in 1985 [31]. This technique consists in inserting a single device with an optical channel and two/three operating channels through the anus. Pneumatic expansion of the rectum is carried out by CO2insufflation . The surgical technique consists in removing the whole rectum wall affected by the carcinoma while maintaining a healthy mucosa margin of at least 5 mm. At the end of removal the rectal wall is sutured [32]. The suture is mandatory in intraperitoneal tumors, where any perforation rapidly transforms into peritonitis, while it is debateable in cases of subperitoneal localization.

Currently this technique is indicated for carcinomas that at the end of clinical-instrumental staging are less than 3 cm in diameter, not ulcerated, Tis or T1 N0 stage and not at "high risk" [33, 34]; in these cases, TEM is safe, with oncological results comparable to those of classic surgery (with five year survival around 85% and a near-zero relapse rate in some studies [34]), and moreover with all the advantages of less invasive surgery.

The type of carcinoma which best suits this type of surgical exeresis is a small, polypoid carcinoma localized in the posterior wall of the subperitoneal rectum, Tis or T1 sm1. Carcinomas considered as "high risk" (in which the relapse rate reaches 23-30% [34]) include all those with one or more of these clinical or histopathological characteristics: submucosa invasion > sm1, grading G3, lymphovascular invasion, mucinous histotype, localization at the last 3 cm of the rectum, resection margins Rx or R1 [33].

In all these cases the evidence-based literature suggests an immediate or delayed (i.e., after the definitive histological exam has been obtained) operation that allows a total excision of the mesorectum.

However, neoadjuvant therapy is increasingly extending the indications of this kind of surgical approach; some early results on carcinomas at a stage greater than T1 are encouraging [25, 34], and it is easy to imagine that the effect of radiotherapy on the primitive tumor and on any lymph-node stations involved can only improve patient outcome, as in radical operations. When we have the results of wider studies currently in progress (UK-TREK) we will be able to better define any expansion of the indications, associating TEM to radiotherapy.

Currently, TEM seems to be a reasonable and safe (in the above-mentioned cases) compromise between resection and the watch and wait approach [35] (devised and experimented by Habr-Gama in carcinomas of the rectum with complete regression after neoadjuvant radiochemiotherapy), feasible in low-stage tumors of the rectum. The microsurgical procedure has the undoubted advantage of permitting a correct staging of the T and a complete exeresis without creating major long-term modifications of the Wexner score or the patient's quality of life [36]. The impossibility of a correct staging of lymph-node involvement currently remains the real weak point in this surgical approach; however, in order to solve this problem studies in progress are assessing the possibility of searching for the sentinel lymphnode inside the mesorectum, by means of scintigraphic marking or vital staining. If the carcinoma removed by TEM should be revealed as being at high risk, the marker will be injected into the scar and the sentinel lymph-node(s) searched for laparoscopically; this will show whether TME is still indicated , once the histological exam has been performed [25].

Even more recent, as we mentioned before, is the appearance of the first study on the transanal approach to rectocolic resection (NOTES), of which TEM is considered the launchpad (from a technical viewpoint and in terms of the instruments required) [37]. The first studies [38] have demonstrated that this technique does not worsen the surgical result in terms of respecting the margins and the number of lymph-nodes. However, in the few cases reported, it is often mandatory to use the classic technique or a laparotomy to permit mobilization of the viscera. Further studies (with short, medium and long term results) and also some technical progress will obviously be necessary to officially consider NOTES as one of the alternatives available in the surgical treatment of rectal cancer.

7.11 Hartmann

We should mention here the famous operation pioneered by Henry Hartmann, remembering that it is currently indicated in treating cancer of the rectum only in cases in which a TME must be performed in seriously incontinent patients, but who are not eligible for abdominoperineal amputation [39].

References

1. Sartori C (2004) Principes generaux sur le positionnement des trocars en chirurgie laparoscopique. “La philosophie du placement des trocarts”. Le Journal de Coelio-Chirurgie 51:35-42
2. Lopez-Kostner F, Lavery IC, Hool GR eta al (1998) Total mesorectal excision is not necessary for cancers of the upper rectum. Surgery 124: 612-618
3. Park IJ, Choi GS, Lim KH et al (2008) Different pattern of lymphatic spread of sigmoid, rectosigmoid and rectal cancers. Ann Surg Oncol 15:3478-3483
4. Heald RJ, Husband EM, Ryall RD (1982) The mesorectum in rectal cancer surgery: the clue to pelvic recurrence? Br J Surg 69:613-616
5. Heald RJ, Smedh RK, Kald A et al (1997) Abdominoperineal excision of the rectum- an endangered operation. Dis Colon Rectum 40:747-751
6. Guillem JG, Chessin DB, Shia J et al (2007) A prospective pathologic analysis using whole-mount sections of rectal cancer following preoperative combined modality therapy. Ann Surg 245:88-93
7. Rullier E, Laurent C, Bretagnol F et al (2005) Sphincter-saving resection for all rectal carcinomas. The end of the 2-cm distal rule. Ann Surg 241:465-469
8. Leo E, Belli F, Miceli R, Mariani L et al (2009) Distal clearance margin of 1 cm or less: a safe distance in lower rectum cancer surgery. Int J colorectal Dis 24:317-322
9. Kusters M, Marijnen CAM, van de Velde CJH (2010) Patterns of local recurrence in rectal cancer; a study of the Dutch TME trial. EJSO 36:470-476

10. Bujko K, Rutkowski A, Chang GJ et al (2012) Is the 1-cm Rule of Distal Bowel Resection Margin in Rectal Cancer Based on Clinical Evidence? A Systematic Review. Ann Surg Oncol 19:801-808
11. van Gijn W, Marijnen CA, Nagtegaal ID (2011) Preoperative radiotherapy combined with total mesorectal excision for resectable rectal cancer: 12-year follow-up of the multicentre, randomised controlled TME trial. Lancet Oncol 12:575-82
12. Pricolo VE, Abodeely A, Resnick M (2010) Distal Margins in Radical Resections for Rectal Cancer after Chemoradiation Therapy: How Short Is Long Enough? Dig Surg 27:185-189
13. Lange MM, Buunen M, van de Velde CJ, Lange JF (2008) Low tie preferred in rectal cancer surgery. Colon Rectum 51:1139-1145
14. Titu LV, Tweedle E, Rooney PS (2008) High Tie of the IMA in curative surgery for left colonic and rectal cancers: a systematic review. Dig Surgery 25:148-157
15. Kanemitsu Y, Hirai T, Komori K, Kato T (2006) Survival benefit of high ligation of the inferior mesenteric artery in sigmoid colon or rectal cancer surgery. Br J Surg 93:609-615
16. Komen N, Slieker J, de Kort P et al (2011) High tie versus low tie in rectal surgery: comparison of anastomotic perfusion. Int J Colorectal Dis 26:1075-1078
17. Nano M, Dal Corso H, Ferronato M et al (2004) Ligation of the inferior mesenteric artery in the surgery of rectal cancer: anatomical considerations. Dig Surg 21:123-6
18. Hashiguchi Y, Hase K, Ueno H et al (2011) Optimal margins and limphadenectomy in colonic cancer surgery. Br J Surg 98: 1171-1178
19. Kang J, Hur H, Min BS et al (2011) Prognostic Impact of Inferior Mesenteric Artery Lymph Node Metastasis in Colorectal Cancer. Ann Surg Oncol 18:704-710
20. Mallassagne B, Valleur P, Serra J et al (1993) Relationship of apical node involvement to serviva in resecate colon carcinoma. Dis Colon Rectum 36: 645-653
21. Heald RJ, Ryall RDH (1986)Recurrence and survival after total mesorectal excision for rectal cancer. The Lancet i:1479-82
22. Ito M, Sugito M, Kobayashi A et al (2008) Relationship between multiple numbers of stapler firings during rectal division and anastomotic leakage after laparoscopic rectal resection. Int J Colorectal Dis 23:703-707
23. Targarona EM, Balague C, Martinez C et al (2008) Laparoscopic low rectal anastomosis using a new stapling device: early experience with the Contour stapler.Minim Invasive Ther Allied Technol 17:155-159
24. Vithiananthan S, Cooper Z, Betten K et al (2001) Hybrid laparoscopic flexure takedown and open procedure for rectal resection is associated with significantly shorter length of stay than equivalent open resection. Dis Colon Rectum 44:927-935
25. Morino M, Verra M, Famiglietti F, Arezzo A (2011) Natural Orifice Transluminal Endoscopic Surgery (NOTES) and colorectal cancer? Colorectal Disease 13:47-50
26. Kim JS, Cho SY, Min BS, Kim NK (2009) Risk factors for anastomotic leakage after laparoscopic intracorporeal colorectal anastomosis with a double stapling technique. J Am Coll Surg 209:694-701
27. West NP, Finan PJ, Anderin C et al (2008) Evidence of the Oncologic Superiority of Cylindrical Abdominoperineal Excision for Low Rectal Cancer. J Clin Oncol 26:3517-3522
28. Holm T, Ljung A, Haggmark T, Jurell G, Lagergren J (2007) Extended abdominoperineal resection with gluteus maximusflap reconstruction of the pelvic floor for rectal cancer. Br J Surg 94:232-238
29. Mauvais F, Sabbagh C, Brehant O (2011) The current abdominoperineal resection: Oncological problems and surgical modifications for low rectal cancer Regimbeau Journal of Visceral Surgery 148:e85-e93
30. Kim JS, Hur H, Kim NK et al (2009) Oncologic Outcomes After Radical Surgery Following Preoperative Chemoradiotherapy for Locally Advanced Lower Rectal Cancer: Abdominoperineal Resection Versus Sphincter-Preserving Procedure Ann Surg Oncol 16:1266-1273
31. Buess G, Theiss R, Gunther M et al (1985) Endoscopic surgery in the rectum. Endoscopy 17:31-35

32. Lezoche G, Guerrieri M, Baldarelli M et al (2011) Transanal endoscopic microsurgery for 135 patients with small nonadvanced low rectal cancer (iT1-iT2, iN0): short- and long-term results. Surg Endosc 25:1222-1229
33. Hompes R, Cunningham C (2011) Extending the role of Transanal Endoscopic Microsurgery (TEM) in rectal cancer Colorectal Disease. The Association of Coloproctology of Great Britain and Ireland 13:32-36
34. Morino M, Allaix ME, Caldart M et al (2011) Risk factors for recurrence after transanal endoscopic microsurgery for rectal malignant neoplasm. Surg Endosc 25:3683-3690
35. Habr-Gama A, Perez RO, Nadalin W et al (2004) Operative versus nonoperative treatment for stage 0 distal rectal cancer following chemoradiation therapy: long-term results. Ann Surg 240: 711-717
36. Allaix ME, Rebecchi F, Giaccone C et al (2011) Long-term functional results and quality of life after transanal endoscopic microsurgery. British Journal of Surgery 98:1635-1643
37. Marks JH (2011) TEM as a Platform for NOTES. J Gastrointest Surg 15:1313-1315
38. Rieder E, Spaun GO, Khajanchee YS (2011) A natural orifice transrectal approach for oncologic resection of the rectosigmoid: an experimental study and comparison with conventional laparoscopy. Surg Endosc. 25:3357-3363
39. Ng KH, Ng DC, Cheung HY et al (2009) Laparoscopic resection for rectal cancers: lessons learned from 579 cases. Ann Surg 249:82-86

Nerve-sparing Technique in Rectal Cancer

8

Simonetta Masaro, Silvia Palmisano, Piera Leon
and Nicolò de Manzini

8.1 Introduction

Attention to nerve identification in rectal cancer surgery began in Japan in the 1970s, but it was an American surgeon [1, 2] between the 1970s and 1980s who proposed a combination of the nerve-sparing principle with the TME technique. The result was the preservation of urogenital function in 90% of the patients treated, without affecting the oncological outcome. Subsequently, the effectiveness, implementation and safety of the technique were confirmed by Moriya's group [3], and the long-term functional results were documented by the famous Dutch TME trial.

The urinary and sexual functions are controlled by nerve endings of the sympathetic system, which originates from the superior hypogastric plexus and from the parasympathetic nerve fibers (the erectile nerves, the pelvic plexus and its branches). The fibers of the sympathetic system are recognized more easily than the parasympathetic component, because it is located much further inside the pelvis. These structures may be damaged during dissection of the mesorectum between the visceral pelvic fascia and the parietal fascia (known as "Heald's holy plane") [4].

Iatrogenous nerve damage during rectal surgery causes urinary and sexual sequelae, which in a recent revision were estimated respectively at between 21 and 44% [5]. Internationally some scores have been recognized as objectively estimating the weight of this kind of complication: the International Prostate Symptom Score (IPSS), the International Index of Erectile Function (IIEF) and the Female Sexual Function Index (FSFI).

S. Palmisano (✉)
Department of Medicine, Surgery and Health Sciences, General Surgery Unit,
Cattinara University Hospital,
Trieste, Italy
e-mail: silvia.palmisano@aots.sanita.fvg.it

N. de Manzini (ed.), *Rectal Cancer*,
Updates in Surgery
DOI: 10.1007/978-88-470-2670-4_8, © Springer-Verlag Italia 2013

Major contributions to this study have been published in the last few years. Sartori´s group demonstrated retrospectively that severe urinary dysfunctions are rare compared to sexual ones, which still represent a problem in terms of reduction of sex drive and spontaneous erectile function, although in 70% of cases adequate orgasmic capacity, penetration and ejaculation are maintained [6].

The male genital function is affected by many factors. Kim and colleagues identified some of these factors, including age above 60 years, low location of rectal cancer, and a follow-up of less than 6 months, as independent risk factors for postoperative sexual dysfunction [7].

An important study on erectile capacity conducted by Song et al. was based on 112 patients treated with TME and nerve preservation. The patients were divided into two groups: one undergoing neoadjuvant radiotherapy followed by surgical treatment (RTS group), and the other treated with surgery alone (Surg group). The IIEF global score had gone down significantly at the post treatment follow-up compared to the initial one in both groups, but the differences were significantly greater in the RTS compared to the Surg group ($p=0.028$). Furthermore, within the RTS group, a statistically significant difference was reported according to the type of surgical operation performed: in patients who had undergone abdominoperineal amputation the erectile function was worse than in those who had had low anterior resection ($p=0.023$).

It has also been demonstrated that radiotherapy has a negative effect on the peripheral nerve fibers, probably due to neurovascular injury, which may also cause muscular atony and atrophy, widespread fibrosis and mucous irritation [8].

The Stamopoulos group also reported other risk factors of nerve damage. Advanced tumors and chemotherapy have resulted in worse IIEF scores, and patient psychology is not the least important aspect of the situation. The mere presence of a colostomy, for instance, may cause a person to feel ashamed of his/her own body, with consequent repercussions on sex life and relationships [9].

8.2 Neuroanatomy and Neurophysiology

8.2.1 Sympathetic System

The sympathetic roots come out of L1, L2 and L3 and make up the *superior hypogastric plexus* located in front of the aorta. They have a left trunk very close to the inferior mesenteric vessels and a deeper right trunk, in the aorto-caval plane (Fig. 8.1). The left trunk runs along the left side of the aorta and towards the end of its route goes past the anterior aortic wall and joins with the right trunk.

The *presacral plexus* at the level of the promontory divides into the right and left *pelvic or hypogastric nerves*, which run parallel and 1-2 cm medially to the ureters (Fig. 8.2).

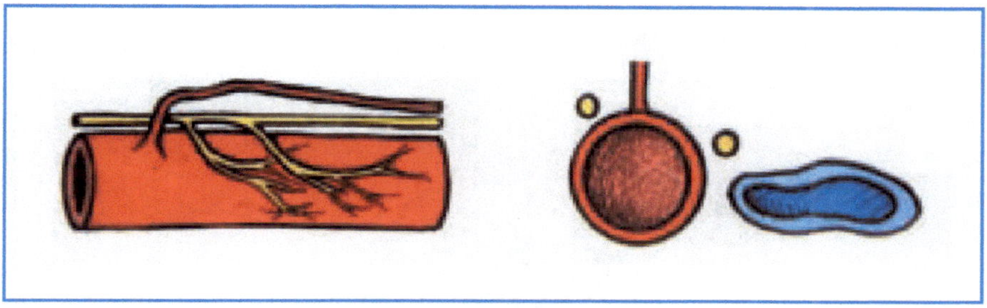

Fig. 8.1 Schematic view of the anatomy of hypogastric nerves along the aorta and crossing the IMA (Inferior Mesenteric Artery)

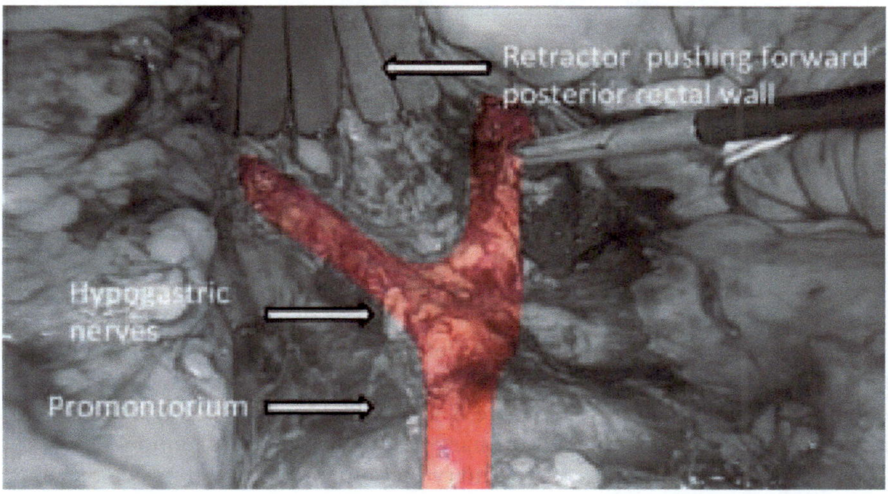

Fig. 8.2 Hypogastric nerves after posterior dissection of fascia recti, pulled forward by the retractor

The *pelvic nerves* run along the postero-superior portion of the mesorectum, externally to the visceral portion of the pelvic fascia and end on each side to form the *inferior hypogastric plexus* or *pelvic plexus*. It is covered and surrounded by the parietal portion of the pelvic fascia.

8.2.2 Parasympathetic System

This is made up of the branches of S2, S3 and S4. The *nervi erigentes* or *cavernous nerves,* in both males and females, run together to the sympathetic branches, externally at the Denonvilliers aponeurosis, behind the anterolateral

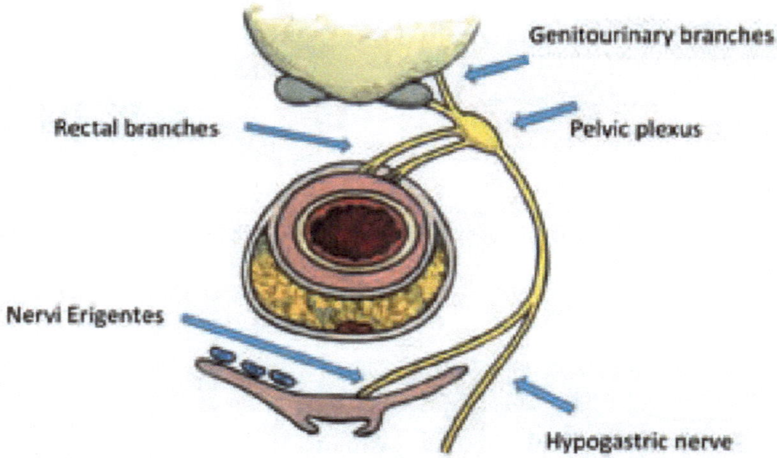

Fig. 8.3 Schematic view of the anatomy of the pelvic nerves and plexi

face of the distal rectum at the seminal vesicles (Walsh neurovascular bundle).

The nerves of the sympathetic system are responsible for urinary continence, and in males they are essential for ejaculation. From a neurophysical viewpoint the internal urethral orifice is innervated by sympathetic signals and has two functions, guaranteeing urinary continence and preventing reflux of sperm during ejaculation. In fact, urinary incontinence and retrograde ejaculation are the results of a failure to preserve the hypogastric nerves bilaterally. The same reason causes an absence of vaginal lubrication in females.

The roots of the parasympathetic nerves at the level of the II-III sacral foramen are responsible for bladder detrusor muscle contraction and for erection. Lesions, according to the number of branches involved, lead to impotence or urinary disturbances, which may reach the denerved bladder [10].

Some nerve fibers originate from ganglion cells of the inferior hypogastric plexus, running from the subperitoneal rectum to the genitourinary organs (Fig. 8.3).

8.3 Sites at Risk

There are four key areas where attention can be focused during this kind of surgery: one in the abdomen and three in the pelvis.

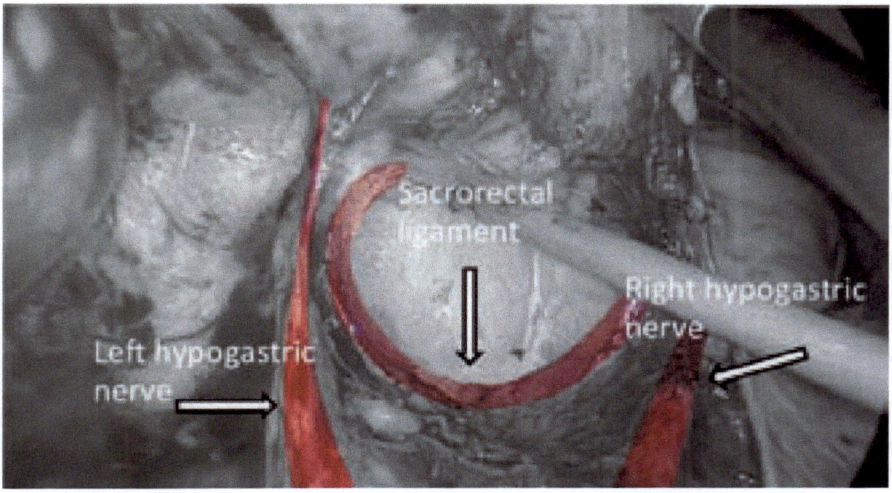

Fig. 8.4 A deeper view of hypogastric nerves crossing the sacrorectal ligament

1. The Origin of the Inferior Mesenteric Artery (IMA): The sympathetic hypogastric nerves are at risk during artery ligature at this point. Damage to the hypogastric plexus or to the hypogastric nerves may cause reduced vesicle compliance, which may lead to emergency incontinence and a lower bladder volume. On the other hand, it has been seen that preserving one side of the plexus clinically results in acceptable urinary continence [11-12]. Furthermore, section of the paraortic trunk may cause erection without ejaculation and/or retrograde ejaculation (the so-called "dry orgasm") [13].

2. Posterior Dissection of the Mesorectum: The nerve endings lie along the deep fascia on the level followed during surgical manoeuvre of presacral dissection. The nerve fibers are easily damaged when the correct plane is not respected. At this level the damage is purely sympathetic (Fig. 8.4).

3. Lateral dissection: This may involve the pelvic plexus and some parasympathetic branches running parallel to it. Radical lymphadenectomy procedures may lead to nerve damage in this area, resulting in sympathetic and parasympathetic complications.

4. Anterior Dissection: During deep dissection of the extraperitoneal rectum anteriorly, behind the prostate and the seminal vesicles, or during hemostasis, the cavernous nerves are at risk. This is where most of parasympathetic

damage occurs, which explains the incidence of greater erectile dysfunction in patients undergoing low pelvic dissection [5].

It has been demonstrated that both fecal and urinary incontinence after treatment for rectal carcinoma are caused by inappropriate movement of the pelvic pavement, or by an inadequate change in the anorectal angle due to a dysfunction of the elevator muscle of the anus, which is not innerved by pudendal nerves, but receives motor fibers from endings which run along its surface. These endings can be destroyed during deep surgical dissection in the pelvis, especially in the case of tumors situated in the low rectum [14].

8.4 Nerve-sparing Technique

It is still an open question as to what is the safest point of the ligature of the inferior mesenteric artery (IMA) and the left paraortic trunk, and the distance between the latter and the origin of the left colic artery. Despite the great variability of the site of the meeting point of the nerve along the IMA, it has been shown that the left paraortic trunk never crosses the artery at its original level. Our conclusion is therefore that the safest point to perform the vascular ligature is within 0.5 cm of the origin of the lower mesenteric artery [13] (Fig. 8.5).

In dissection at the level of the pelvis, if the TME principle is rigorously followed it is possible to minimize the risk of iatrogenous lesions of the pelvic nerve endings of the autonomous system, including the innervation of the anal elevator muscle (Fig. 8.6).

In spite of the fact that dissection in front of Denonvilliers' fascia was described by Heald as the best oncological procedure [15], other authors have preferred a dissection behind this fascia as the best way of guaranteeing the safety of the nerves of the autonomous system, and consequently the urogenital functions [16]. On the other hand, the Lindsey group recommends an approach tailored to individual patients, performing dissection in front of Denonvilliers' fascia only in the event of anterior carcinomas [17].

An instrument for intraoperative nerve identification has recently been introduced. The effectiveness of a nerve stimulator to identify nerves recurring bilaterally is already known in the field of thyroid surgery. The same concept has been applied to rectal surgery, with the use of the Cavermap® to identify or confirm nerve structures in the pelvis in the event of uncertainty. The Da Silva group enrolled 29 sexually active male patients subjected to elective TME for rectal cancer, and applied to them the nerve stimulator and a sensor of erectile response for intraoperative use. The study showed good results in terms of determination of both the hypogastric and the cavernous nerves, with their preservation in 93% of cases and without reported adverse effects connected to the use of this instrument [18].

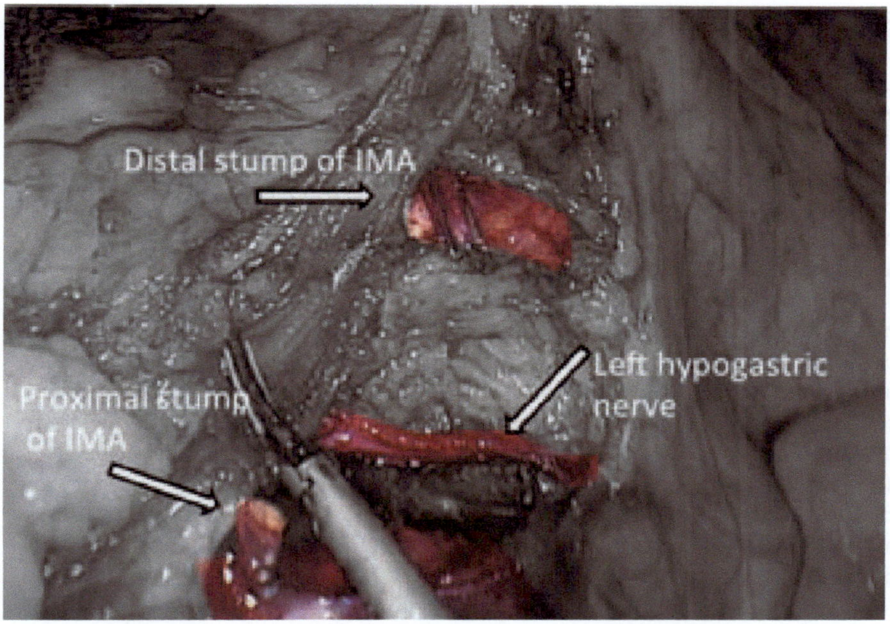

Fig. 8.5 Left hypogastric nerve as it appears after section of the IMA at its origin

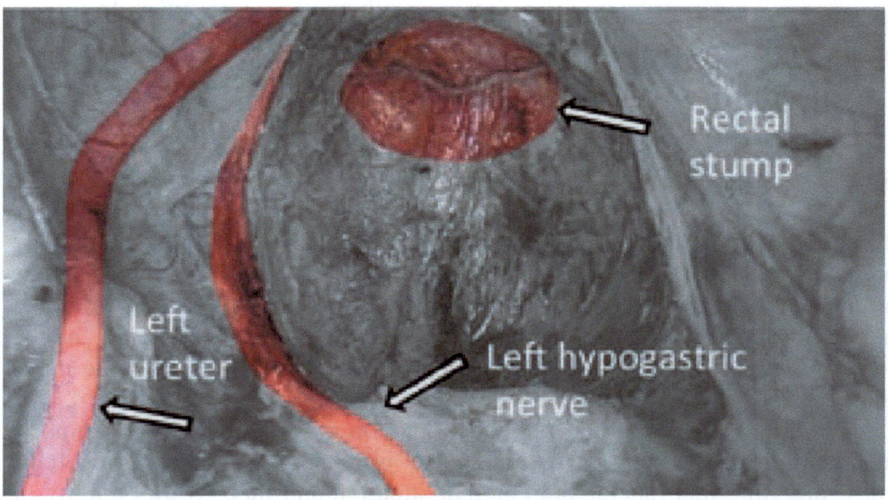

Fig. 8.6 After specimen removal, ureter, hypogastric nerve and rectal stump are visible in the empty pelvis

8.5 Role of Laparoscopy

Laparoscopic rectal surgery offers a significant advantage as regards safeguarding postoperative sexual functions. This advantage may be attributed to the improvement in intraoperative vision provided by optical magnification, and the use of the 30° view, which characterizes this approach. In fact, it has been demonstrated that since the introduction of laparoscopic surgery, there has been no increase either in sexual dysfunctions or vesicle functions acquired after surgery [19-20].

As regards the incidence of sexual dysfunctions after treatment for rectal carcinoma, we can cite a prospective study carried out by a Greek group. This compares the effects of laparoscopy and traditional open surgery. Stamopoulos and his colleagues studied 56 patients, all of whom were male and underwent rectal surgery for cancer, demonstrating that the IIEF went down significantly in the postoperative period ($p<0.01$) in both groups. They did not observe any significant differences between the group undergoing laparoscopic surgery and the one undergoing open surgery, but there was a trend favoring laparoscopy at the 6-month follow up. The IIEF score in the immediate postoperative period, at 3 and at 6 months, was better in patients subjected to anterior low resection compared to the group undergoing abdominoperineal amputation. Tumors T3 and T4 registered lower scores ($p=0.001$) [9].

The retrospective study by Morino's group shows that laparoscopic TME does not lead to better outcomes than good surgery performed with open technique, in terms of sexual and urinary functions. A transient urinary dysfunction is recorded in 14% of patients, all treated with medical therapy alone. Patients who underwent anterior resection developed a significant deficit of erection in 23.7%, while in 71.4% ($p=0.039$) after abdomino-perineal amputation [21].

8.6 Conclusions

To conclude, postsurgical nerve damage and, to a lesser extent, radiotherapy are the main factors in the etiology of the dysfunction of the pelvic organs after rectal cancer treatment. Systematically identifying and safeguarding the nerves during surgery are therefore essential. Ligature at the origin of the lower mesenteric artery and rigorous adherence to the TME technique minimize the risk of iatrogenous nerve lesions.

It is important to highlight how dysfunction of the pelvic organs impacts negatively on the patient on several levels, physically as well as psychologically, affecting their social and emotive situation and their overall quality of life [14].

References

1. Hojo K, Vernava A (1991) Preservation of urine voiding and sexual function after rectal cancer surgery. Dis Colon Rectum 34:532-539
2. Enker WE (1992) Potency, cure, and local control in the operative treatment of rectal cancer. Arch Surg 127:1396-1401
3. Maas CP, Moriya Y, Steup WH et al (2000) A prospective study on radical and nerve-preserving surgery for rectal cancer in the Netherlands. Eur J Surg Oncol 26:751-757
4. Celentano V et al (2010) Prospective study of sexual dysfunction in men with rectal cancer: feasibility and results of nerve sparing surgery. Int J Colorectal Dis 25:1441-1445
5. Lindsey I (2000) Anatomy of Denonvilliers' fascia and pelvic nerves, impotence, and implications for the colorectal surgeon. Br J Surg 87:1288-1299
6. Sartori C (2011) Urinary and sexual disorders after laparoscopic TME for rectal cancer in males. J Gastrointest Surg 15:637-643
7. Kim et al (2002) Assessment of sexual and voiding function after total mesorectal excision with pelvic autonomic nerve preservation in males with rectal cancer. Dis Colon Rectum 45:1178-1185
8. Song PH et al (2010) Comparison of the erectile function in male patients with rectal cancer treated by preoperative radiotherapy followed by surgery and surgery alone. Int J Colorectal Dis 25:619-624
9. Stamopoulos P et al (2009) Prospective evaluation of sexual function after open and laparoscopic surgery for rectal cancer. Surg Endosc 23:2665-2674
10. de Calan L, Gayet B, Bourlier P et al (2004) Cancer du rectum: anatomie chirurgicale, preparation à l'intervention, installation du patient. In: Encyclopédie Médico-Chirurgicale 40-606 Editions Scientifiques et Médicales Elseviers, Paris, pp 1-12
11. Matsuoka N, Moriya Y, Akasu T et al (2001) Long-term outcome of urinary function after extended lymphadenectomy in patients with distal rectal cancer. Eur J Surg Oncol 27:165-169
12. Moriya Y (2006) Function preservation in rectal cancer surgery. Int J Clin Oncol 11:339-343
13. Nano M et al (2004) Ligation of the Inferior Mesenteric Artery in the surgery of rectal cancer: anatomical considerations. Dig Surg 21:123-127
14. Lange MM, van de Valde CJH (2010) Long-term anorectal and urogenital dysfunction after rectal cancer treatment. Semin Colon Rectal Surg 21:87-94
15. Heald RJ et al (2004) Optimal total mesorectal excision for rectal cancer is by dissection in front of Denonvilliers' fascia. Br J Surg 91:121-123
16. Kinugasa Y et al (2006) Operating behind Denonvilliers' fascia for reliable preservation of urogenital autonomic nerves in total mesorectal excision. A histologic study using cadaveric specimens, including a surgical experiment using fresh cadaveric models. Dis Colon Rectum 49:1024-1032
17. Lindsey I et al (2005) Denonvilliers' fascia lies anterior to the fascia propria and rectal dissection plane in total mesorectal excision. Dis Colon Rectum 48:37-42
18. Da Silva G (2004) The efficacy of a nerve stimulator (Cavermap®) to enhance autonomic nerve identification and confirm nerve preservation during total mesorectal excision. Dis Colon Rectum 47:2032-2038
19. Asoglu O et al (2009) Impact of laparoscopic surgery on bladder and sexual function after total mesorectal excision for rectal cancer. Surg Endosc 23:296-303
20. Breukink SO et al (2005) Laparoscopic versus open total mesorectal excision: a case-control study. Int J colorectal Dis 20:428-433
21. Morino M, Parini U, Allaix ME et al (2009) Male sexual and urinary function after laparoscopic total mesorectal excision. Surg Endosc 23:1233-1240

References

Reconstruction

9

Paola Tarchi, Elisa Moretti and Nicolò de Manzini

9.1 Colorectal and Coloanal Anastomosis

At present, preservation of the anal sphincter is possible in the majority of low rectal (LR) carcinomas; indeed, by associating neoadjuvant radiochemotherapy (RCT) to TME, it is possible to preserve the sphincter in at least 70% of cases [1]. However, it is obvious that proctectomy, followed by straight coloanal or colorectal anastomosis (SCA), significantly modifies the mechanisms of continence and defecation. The functional results after anterior resection (AR) in low resections (LAR) with direct anastomosis (end-to-end), located less than 10 cm from the anal margin and in absence of preoperative radiotherapy, report good continence rates in just 20% of cases, against 100% of high AR (Fig. 9.1) [2].

In fact, in LAR the rectum's function as a storage tank is eliminated or significantly reduced, and the activity of the sphincter is frequently impaired, while changes to the external sphincter and the pelvic floor are less frequent Thus 5% of patients present incontinence, 60% soiling or important modifications of the bowel movements, 16% require incontinence pads, 63.2% are unable to discern gas from feces, and 18% are constipated. This state of affairs has been given the name "anterior resection syndrome" (ARS), which can be summarized by the presence of frequency, urgency, fragmentation and incontinence to feces [3]. The result is a profound change in the quality of life, making it impossible to carry on working and lead a normal social life.

In an attempt to improve postoperative functionality, which is also affected by any neoadjuvant radiotherapy [4], three one-stage surgical reconstruc-

P. Tarchi (✉)
Department of Medicine, Surgery and Health Sciences, General Surgery Unit,
Cattinara University Hospital,
Trieste, Italy
e-mail: paolatarchi@hotmail.com

N. de Manzini (ed.), *Rectal Cancer,*
Updates in Surgery
DOI: 10.1007/978-88-470-2670-4_9, © Springer-Verlag Italia 2013

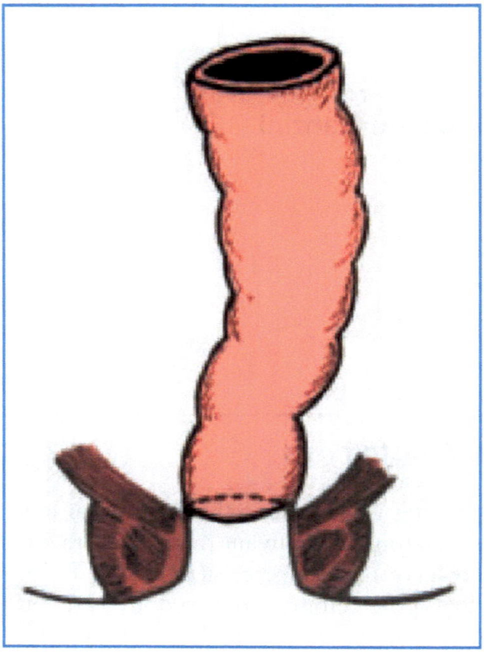

Fig. 9.1 Straight coloanal anastomosis

tion techniques have been proposed as an alternative to SC: colonic J-pouch, coloplasty and side-to-end anastomosis. Debate is on-going about which reconstruction technique is best in terms of functionality, low postoperative morbidity and quality of life.

The creation of a reservoir would appear to be useful in terms of better functional results for anastomoses less than 8 cm from the anal margin, according to the comparative study by Hida [5], whereas in Montesani's [6] case study, the reference cut-off is 6 cm from the anal margin. In our Institute we perform reconstruction with anastomotic reservoir for cancer located at less than 5 cm from the anal margin and in coloanal anastomosis. The creation of a colic reservoir during coloanal anastomosis for low rectal cancer is undoubtedly a uniformly recommended standard in clinical practice [7].

The first reconstruction technique was the colonic J-pouch, proposed by Lazorthes [8] and Parc [9] in 1986; the idea was to create a reservoir to make up for the loss of the rectal compliance function by using the sigma folded and anastomosed laterally on itself and latero-terminally, on its apex, at the anus or at the residual portion of the rectum (Fig. 9.2) [10]. The optimum size of the colonic J-pouch would seem to be 5-7 cm [11]. The volume of the neo-ampulla established in this way varies between 250 and 350 cc, and anastomosis to the anus is performed manually with the most distal part of the pouch. In cases of widespread sigmoid diverticulitis, the descending colon is generally used, prior to ample mobilization of the left colonic flexure.

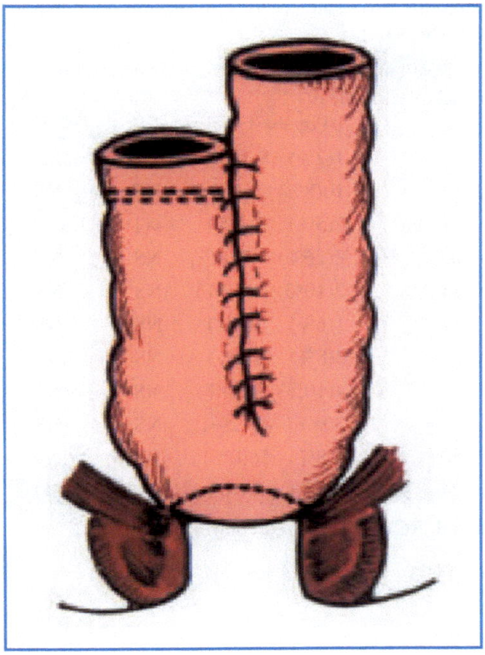

Fig. 9.2 Colonic J-pouch

Electrophysiological studies carried out recently appear to indicate that the pouch's tank function, rather than its tank shape, is connected to the local segmental denervation subsequent to the opening of the colonic wall, which determines a slowing of fecal transit in the immediately supra-anastomotic area.

A study performed by the Cleveland Clinic [12] demonstrated that the reconstruction of intestinal continuity using the J-pouch is possible in the majority of cases. It was not possible in 26.1% of patients for 5 technical reasons: primarily the presence of a narrow pelvis (42.9%), followed by finding a large pelvic muscular mass or the need for partial resection of the internal sphincter and/or mucosectomy and/or manual anastomosis (32.2%), by concomitant diffused diverticular disease (10.7%), by insufficient length of the colon to move down (7.1%), and finally by pregnancy (3.6%).

Data from Heriot's [13] meta-analysis illustrated the short-term complications between J-pouch and SCA: the average anastomotic leak rate was 13% in SCA versus 9% in the J-pouch group; 7% of anastomotic strictures was observed in both groups; the paper also reports 7% of wound infections and 2% of recto-vaginal fistula in both groups. Overall morbidity and mortality were comparable, with no statistically significant difference between J-pouch and SCA (0% vs. 1-2%). Several trials investigated the surgical outcome of these two reconstruction techniques, especially in terms of fistula formation, confirming no difference in postoperative complications (Table 9.1). The main difference between SCA and J-pouch concerns the early functional results:

Table 9.1 Trials investigating the rates of anastomotic leaks and strictures in patients operated on for J-pouch versus straight coloanal anastomosis (SCA)

Author	Year	Study type	No. of patients J-Pouch/S.C.A.	Anastomotic leak J-Pouch/SCA	Anastomotic stricture J-Pouch/SCA
Hallbook [14]	1996	RCT	45 52	1(2%) 8(15%)	NS NS
Dehni [15]	1998	R	122 136	10(8%) 21(15%)	NS NS
Prete [16]	2000	RCT	35 31	2(5%) 2(6%)	4(11%) 3(9%)
Willis [17]	2001	PRN	31 63	8(26%) 15(24%)	NS NS
Gotzinger [18]	2001	PRN	20 25	2(10%) 3(12%)	NS NS
Mantyh [19]	2001	PRN	16 17	1(6%) 1(6%)	NS NS
Furst [20]	2002	RCT	37 37	3(8%) 1(3%)	NS NS
Lin [21]	2002	PRN	40 41	4(10%) 4(10%)	NS NS
Sailer [22]	2002	RCT	32 32	3(9%) 4(12%)	NS NS
Machado [23, 24]	2003 (2005)	RCT	50 50	4(8%) 5(10%)	1(2%) 2(4%)
Jiang [25]	2005	RCT	24 24	1(4%) 0(0%)	0(0%) 1(4%)

R, randomized; *PRN*, prospective non-randomized; *RCT*, randomized controlled trial.

patients with J-pouch tend to have less frequency, urgency and difficulty in evacuation immediately after surgery and up to 1 year after the operation.

The use of an alternative technique such as coloplasty (Fig.9.3) has reduced the number of cases in which SCA was necessary to 5.3% [12]. This reconstruction technique, which is designed to interrupt the antegrade colonic peristalsis, consists in performing a longitudinal section of approximately 7-10 cm along the anterior wall of the lowered colon approximately 4 cm from the site of the manual or stapled direct colorectal or coloanal anastomosis, then suturing it transversally, following the classic Heinecke-Mikulicz [26, 27] pyloroplasty technique. Most of the studies published report complications and similar early postoperative functional results between transversal coloplasty and J-pouch. The randomized clinical trial by Ulrich et al. [26] compared 73 J-pouch to 76 coloplasty cases (systemic loop ileostomy): the anastomotic leak rate was 8% in both groups, with pelvic sepsis developing in 3% of J-pouch vs. 1% of coloplasty cases. Postoperative mortality was null in both groups. Another study [27] conducted on a smaller cohort of patients (12 coloplasty and 35 J-pouch, again all with loop ileostomy) reported no significant difference in the outcome of the two groups; specifically, the early functional results assessed through the Wexner score 1 year after surgery gave a score of 6 in the coloplasty and 7 in the J-pouch cases.

A further alternative technique, proposed as early as 1950, is the "side-to-end anastomosis" (Fig. 9.4), created manually or mechanically about 3 cm from the terminal suture of the colon [28]. This blind segment was devised to act as a mini-pouch; in reality it seems to work simply by slowing the distal

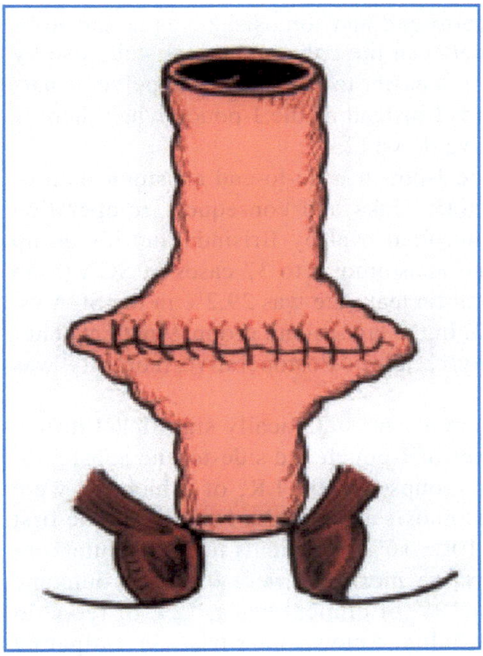

Fig.9.3 Coloplasty

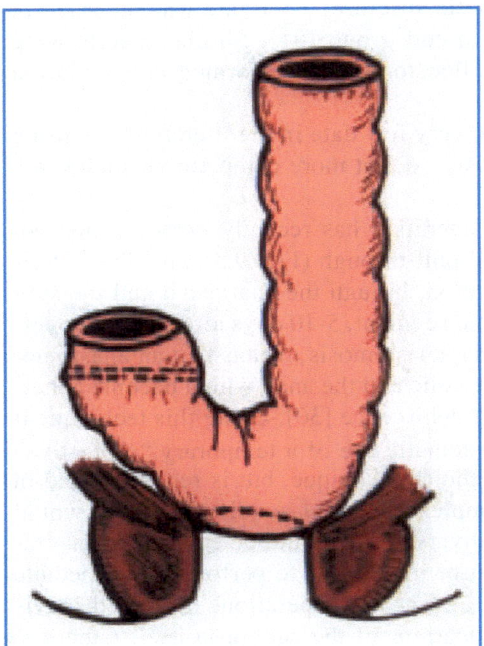

Fig. 9.4 Side-to-end anastomosis

colic movement [23, 29, 30]. The side-to-end anastomosis solves major problems related to the different calibre between the colic and rectal stub, also by minimising the size of the reservoir; it is easier to perform if the pelvis is narrow. Finally, it is strongly recommended instead of the J-pouch when there is insufficient length of the colon to move down [23].

As previously demonstrated for the J-pouch, side-to-end anastomosis promotes a lower incidence of anastomotic leaks and consequent re-operation compared to SCA. A randomized controlled trial by Brisinda and his group [29] compared 40 cases of side-to-end anastomosis to 37 cases of SCA (loop ileostomy not performed): the anastomotic leak rate was 29.2% in the SCA vs. 5% in the end-to-end group (p=0.005). In the end-to-end group, 9 patients later needed reintervention with colostomy creation. Postoperative mortality was comparable.

On the other hand, once again there are no statistically significant differences in terms of the surgical outcomes of J-pouch and side-to-end anastomosis. Machado [23] randomized two groups of 100 LR, of which 50 were reconstructed with a side-to-end anastomosis and 50 with J-pouch. In the first group the anastomotic leak rate was 10%, 16% of patients needed reintervention, wound infection and post-operative mortality were 0%. The outcome was comparable in the J-pouch group: 8% of clinical leaks, 12% of reoperations, 2% of wound infection and mortality. Among other trials investigating anastomotic leak rates there was no significant heterogeneity: approximately 5% rate of leaks formation in the J-pouch and 2% in the side-to-end group [31]; analyzing the rates of anastomotic stricture, a 5% rate was recorded in the J-pouch versus 6% in the side-to-end group [31]. Similar results were obtained even when a selective loop ileostomy was performed in association with the LAR [25].

Apart from these results, there are very few data in the literature regarding the outcome of side-to-end anastomosis, so that more comparative studies are needed.

An old two-stage reconstructive operation has recently been reproposed: the Turnbull-Cutait abdominoperineal pull-through (Fig. 9.5 a, b). The exteriorization of approximately 8 cm of colon through the anal canal and the subsequent resection of the excess external segment, 5-10 days after the first operation, with manual end-to-end coloanal anastomosis, means that an anastomosis can be created on two surfaces, the colic and the anal, which become adherent and therefore have a lower risk of dehiscence [30]. Using this technique it is possible to avoid or reduce the systematic use of a temporary "protective" ileostomy. This is clearly not a first choice technique, but is recommended in selected patients with extremely complex anorectal conditions which would otherwise require a permanent fecal diversion. It should be considered in situations where it is technically difficult or impossible to perform an immediate coloanal anastomosis, such as in the event of reoperation, irradiated pelvis with chronic inflammation, or complications of the neoplasia itself (stenosis, abscesses, rectovaginal fistulas); it can also be used in patients who categori-

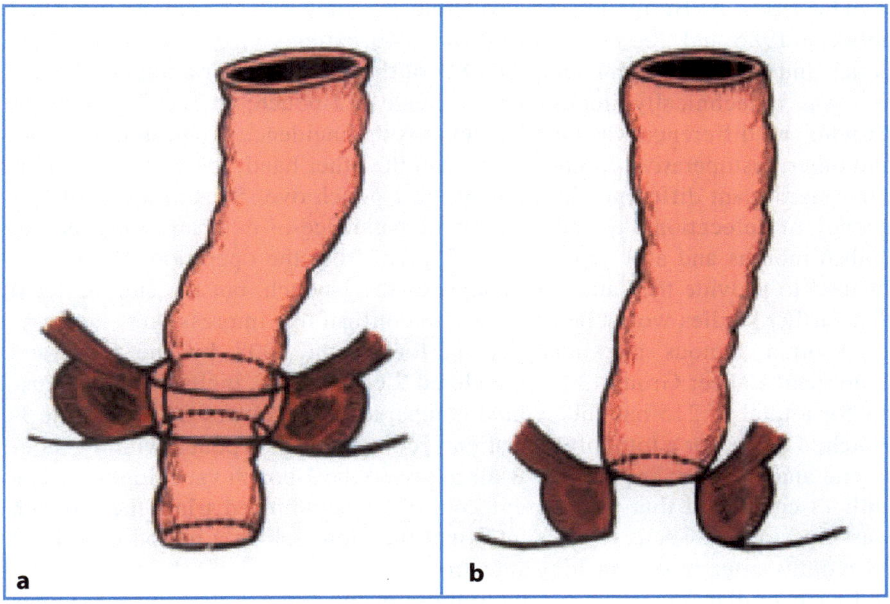

Fig. 9.5 a, b First and second steps of abdominal pull-through. The second step is delayed until 5-10 days after the first operation

cally refuse an ostomy or in severely obese patients in whom the creation of an ostomy is technically difficult due to the thickness of the abdominal wall.

A comparison of the postoperative and long-term results of immediate direct coloanal anastomosis with results of deferred anastomosis on the basis of pull-through operation time does not show any statistically significant differences, except for the incidence of abscesses and anastomotic dehiscence, which appears lower with the pull-through in a study by Remzi et al. [32]. In this paper the authors compared 67 pull-through with 88 SCA cases, with a median follow up of 5.6 years. Anastomotic leak was 7% and 5% ($p=0.048$) respectively; anastomotic strictures 16% and 13%; intra-abdominal abscesses 0% and 5% ($p=0.043$); a trans-anal prolapsus was observed in 7% of pull-through cases. Finally, the long-term median Wexner score was 10.6 in the pull-through vs. 12.2 in the SCA group.

Analysis of the surgical outcome of these reconstruction techniques and comparisons among them has been reviewed in several literature studies, with an unanimous result in stating the absence of a significant difference between incidences of anastomotic leaks between SCA, J-pouch and coloplasty. However, 3 meta-analyses were performed to comparatively assess numerically important cases, and the immediate and long-term functional results of the reconstruction techniques proposed after anterior resection for extraperitoneal rectal carcinoma (medium and low) [13, 31, 33].

The first, by Heriot [13], considered 35 comparative studies published between 1986 and 2005, for a total of 2,240 patients (1,066 SCA, 1,050 J-pouch and 124 coloplasty). Only in 4.8% of the cases, and for a total of 7 studies, was it technically impossible to create a J-pouch; in the 3 groups of patients, no difference was noted as regards the incidence of anastomotic leak and other postoperative complications. On the other hand, there was a statistically significant difference in favor of the J-pouch over SCA in terms of frequency of defecation/day and in terms of incidence of defecatory urgency at both 6 months and at 1 year and at >2 years from the operation. Coloplasty seemed to provide the same advantages as the J-pouch, but the author stated that further studies would be necessary to confirm this impression.

Another famous meta-analysis, performed in 2008 by the Cochrane Colorectal Cancer Group [33], considered 2,609 studies, including only 9 trials for a total of 215 patients, which compared the results of SCA with the J-pouch; 4 trials, for a total of 215 patients, compared the J-pouch with the side-to-end anastomosis; and lastly 3 trials assessed the J-pouch vs. coloplasty. The authors concluded that in different controlled randomized trials the J-pouch was superior to SCA as regards intestinal function and for a period of at least 18 months after re-establishing intestinal continuity. Coloplasty and side-to-end gave similar functional results to those of the J-pouch, but further studies were required to determine the precise role of these alternative reconstructive strategies.

The last meta-analysis, published in 2010 by Siddiqui [31] focused on studies comparing the J-pouch with side-to-end anastomosis between 1980 and 2009, and included 4 randomized controlled trials, for a total of 273 patients (138 J-pouch vs. 135 side-to-end anastomosis). No statistically significant difference emerged between the two techniques in terms of postoperative morbidity and mortality. As regards functional results, statistically significant comparisons were represented by lower basal anal pressure 24 months after the operation, with J-pouch, and lower defecatory incidence at 6 months, in the same group of patients. The authors concluded by stating that both techniques appear safe and have acceptable results, although a controlled randomized trial including several patients would be necessary to highlight this evidence.

9.2 Anoperineal Reconstruction Methods

Over the last ten years, the diffusion of sphincter preservation techniques and of total excision of the mesorectum [34], the application of neoadjuvant therapy, and the clear definition of distal resection margins [35], have reduced the need for abdominoperineal amputation according to Miles in favor of sphincter saving techniques. The Miles operation has a high complication rate, often correlated to the perineal wound (recurrent perineal infection, pelvic abscess, delay in healing, secondary dehiscence), and significantly changes the quality of life of the patients, necessitating an iliac colostomy (IC).

Perineal colostomy (PC) was used for years after Miles' operation to re-establish gastrointestinal continuity; the primary purpose of this technique was to reduce the invalidity deriving from an iliac colostomy in selected and motivated patients capable of managing often daily colonic irrigations. The functional results and the quality of life of patients undergoing this type of reconstruction are comparable to those obtained after IC or coloanal anastomosis [36-39]; furthermore, the presence of a perineal colostomy reduces morbidity at a perineal level as well as the healing time of the wound, especially in patients undergoing neoadjuvant therapy [40].

In the past, numerous procedures were proposed for the reconstruction of the perineal region after the Miles operation [41], which are now no longer used. Initially, Schmidt [42] proposed continent colostomy, which consisted of using a 10-15 cm ring of mucosa removed from the surgical specimen and arranged as a sleeve around terminal portion of the colon. The same technique, using smooth muscle for the perineal colostomy, was performed by Federov [43] with good functional results. Gamagami et al. confirmed these results by achieving continence of 59% of patients with perineal colostomy and free colonic muscle graft after 12 months' follow-up [39].

The use of muscular transposition techniques came after this. These involve autologous perineal plasty using the gluteus maximus muscle, or more frequently the gracilis muscle, to construct a neosphincter. Single or double graciloplasty, initially described by Pickrell for treating children affected by neurogenic fecal incontinence, when associated to perineal colostomy becomes an integral part of the total perineal reconstruction. The quality of the results obtained after graciloplasty depends on the treatment the patient is given in the postoperative rehabilitation process. The few case studies published indicate an improvement of 50% in medium term patients, no matter which muscular transposition is performed [44-46].

Experimental [47] and clinical [48] studies have demonstrated how the result of muscular transpositions could be significantly improved by subjecting the transposed muscles to continual electric stimulation. When this procedure is used, the striated muscles normally subject to fatigue and capable of rapid but short contractions transform into permanent contraction muscles, thanks to an implanted and programmable neurostimulator. In patients subjected to dynamic graciloplasty a restoration of continence is described in 54-83% of cases. Postoperative complications are, however, frequent (described in 40-90% of cases) and explain the observed failures: transplant infection favored by ischemia, ulceration of the anal canal due to excessive tension of the transplant, disinsertion of the tendon implant on the ilium, secondary muscular stimulation defect with rupture or movement of the electrodes [49-51]. The failure of the technique may also be functional and not concern anal continence but rectal evacuation, with the impossibility of a complete emptying in the absence of a daily evacuative enema [52-55].

The most recent option for creating a sphincteral mechanism after abdominoperineal amputation and perineal colostomy consists in implanting (during the same operation or in a second one) an artificial sphincter around the perineal stoma. This technique, initially proposed for treating fecal incontinence in adults, has obtained encouraging results in total anorectal reconstruction; the most recent cases are, however, heterogeneous and extremely few. In particular, Romano et al. [56] describe the implantation of an artificial anal sphincter in 8 patients (synchronous in 5 patients, in two stages in the other 3) undergoing anoperineal reconstruction between 1999 and 2001, reporting one wound infection and three patients with altered evacuation amongst the complications. In the Marchal et al. [57] case studies, implantation of the artificial sphincter was carried out in two operations, in the absence of local or remote recurrence of illness or local sequelae of radiotherapy; of the three patients undergoing the implant, one had wound bruising. In both studies, despite the fact that they were preliminary and numerically limited, this technique showed reduced morbidity compared with graciloplasty, reporting good results in terms of fecal continence and quality of life.

Antegrade colonic irrigation techniques can be recommended only when sphincter replacing techniques are not possible or have proved to be ineffective. The principle behind these techniques envisages a complete intestinal emptying at regular intervals using enemas introduced by a proximal colostomy, which should also be continent, so as to avoid losses or require application of a bag. Several accesses to the proximal colon have been described and tested on a small series of patients: appendicostomy, cecal tube with antireflux system [58], ileum or terminal [59], or even Roux-en-Y anastomosis with the right colon, whose end is grafted to the skin [60].

Among these, appendicostomy, initially described by Malone [61] and recommended in cases of infantile incontinence caused by neurological conditions like spina bifida, Hirschsprung disease or anorectal deformations, was subsequently used also for post-traumatic or neurological incontinence in adults. In 2005, Penninckx et al. [62] and Portier et al. [37] introduced an alternative to total perineal reconstruction (TPR) by associating appendicostomy to perineal colostomy in the absence of graciloplasty, with good results in terms of continence (the Wexner score achieved in the 18 patients of Portier's case study is 6.5/20). The long-term total perineal reconstruction results with dynamic graciloplasty associated to appendicostomy according to Malone have also been encouraging in terms of restoring functionality and quality of life: in Abbes Orabi's [63] study of 10 patients undergoing this procedure and followed up for 78 months, the mortality rate correlated to the procedure was 0, with minimum postoperative morbidity. However, there was a significant rate of late complications (mucosal prolapse and stenosis of the coloperineal anastomosis, stenosis of the graciloplasty and of the appendicostomy, vaginal stenosis), requiring local revision in 13 cases and abdominal re-operation in one case.

Comparison of the functional results reported in literature for the various perineal reconstruction techniques is made difficult by the great heterogeneity exisiting in terms of surgical technique, execution time, number of samples and assessment methods.

9.3 Conclusions

In conclusion, the literature data show how reconstruction with good functional results can be obtained in at least 75% of cases [4] of extraperitoneal rectal cancer. A reconstruction technique with colonic pouch seems to be the best option for all low colorectal anastomoses, and is almost obligatory for coloanal ones. The colonic J-pouch is the most widely tested technique, although it does not seem to provide any different results from coloplasty and from side-to-end anastomosis. The latter two techniques represent valid alternatives to the J-pouch if this is technically either difficult or impossible to perform. The pull-through technique, although used by some centres as the intervention of choice, should be reserved primarily for cases involving complications subsequent to a pouch reconstruction; in this case it represents the last option before a permanent ostomy [25, 30, 31].

The most recent option for reconstruction of the perineal region after a Miles' operation consists in implanting an artificial sphincter around the perineal colostomy [56, 57], which has obtained encouraging results, but is actually performed only in very few centres. Antegrade colonic irrigation by proximal stoma remains the last resort, if the other reconstruction techniques are not successful.

References

1. Heald RJ, Smedh RK, Kald A et al (1997) Abdominoperineal excision of the rectum- an endangered operation. Dis Colon Rectum 40:747-751
2. Batignani G, Monaci I, Ficari F, Tonelli F (1991) What affects continence after anterior resection of the rectum? Dis Colon Rectum 34:329-335
3. Pala C, Serventi F, Paliogiannis P (2009) Le sequel funzionali dopo chirurgia del retto basso. Ann Ital Chir 80:193-197
4. Lange MM, den Dulk M, Bossema ER et al (2007) Risk factors for fecal incontinence after rectal cancer treatment. Br J Surg 94:1278-1284
5. Hida J, Yasutomi M, Maruyama T et al (1998) Indications for colonic J-pouch recostruction after anterior resection for rectal cancer: determing the optimum level of anastomosis. Dis Colon Rectum 41:558-563
6. Montesani C, Pronio A, Santella S et al (2004) Rectal cancer surgery with sphincter preservation: functional results related to the level of anastomosis. Clinical and instrumental study. Hepatogastroenterology 51:718-721
7. Alves A (2007) Reccomendations for clinical practice. Therapeutic choices for rectal cancer. How can we reduce therapeutic sequelae and preserve quality of life? Gastroenterol Clin Biol 31:1S52-62,1S95-7
8. Lazorthes F, Fages P, Chiotasso P et al (1986) Resection of the rectum with costruction of a colonic reservoir and colo-anal anastomosis for carcinoma of the rectum. Br J Surg 73:136-138
9. Parc R, Tiret E, Frileux P et al (1986) Resection and colo-anal anastomosis with colonic reservoir for rectal carcinoma. Br J Surg 73:139-141
10. de la Fuente SG, Mantih CR (2007) Reconstruction techniques after proctectomy: what's the best? Clin Colon and Rectal Surg 20:221-230
11. Dehni N, Parc N (2003) Colonic J-Pouch-Anal Anastomosis for Rectal Cancer. Dis Colon Rectum 46:668-675

12. Harris GJC, Lavery IJ, Fazio VW (2002) Reasons for failure to construct the colonic J-pouch. What can be done to improve the size of the neorectal reservoir Should it occur? Dis Colon Rectum 45:1304-1308
13. Heriot AG, Tekkis PP, Constantinides V et al (2006) Meta-analysis of colonic reservoirs versus straight coloanal anastomosis after anterior resection. Br J Surg 93:19-32
14. Hallbook O, Pahlman L, Krog M et al (1996) Randomized comparison of straight and colonic J pouch anastomosis after low anterior resection. Ann Surg 224:58-65
15. Dehni N, Tiret E, Singland JD et al (1998) Long-term functional outcome after low anterior resection: comparison of low colorectal anastomosis and colonic J-pouch-anal anastomosis. Dis Colon Rectum 41:817-822
16. Prete F, Liguori P, Nitti P et al (2000) Optimal reconstruction after resection of the rectum in cancer surgery. Chir Ital 52:323-328
17. Willis S, Kasperk R, Braun J, Schumpelick V (2001) Comparison of colonic J-pouch reconstruction and straight coloanal anastomosis after intersphincteric rectal resection. Langenbecks arc Surg 386:193-199.
18. Gotzinger P, Wamser P, Herbst F (2001) Colo-anal anastomosis: improvement of early function outcome by reconstruction with the colonic pouch. Chirurg 72:49-53
19. Mantyh CR, Hull TL, Fazio VW (2001) Coloplasty in low colorectal anastomosis: manometric and functional comparison with straight and colonic J-pouch anastomosis. Dis Colon Rectum 44:37-42
20. Furst A, Burghofer K, Hutzel L, Jauch K-W (2002) Neorectal reservoir is not the functional principle of the colonic J-pouch: the volume of a short colonic J-pouch does not differ from a straight coloanal anastomosis. Dis Colon Rectum 45:660-667
21. Lin J-K, Wang H-S, Yang S-H et al (2002) Comparison between straight and J-pouch coloanal anastomosis in surgery for rectal cancer. Surg Today 32:487-492
22. Sailer M, Fuchs KH, Fein M, Thiede A (2002) Randomized clinical trial comparing quality of life after straight and pouch coloanal reconstruction. Br J Surg 89:1108-1117
23. Machado M, Nygren J, Goldman S, Ljungquist O (2003) Similar outcome after colonic pouch and side-to-end anastomosis in low anterior resection for rectal cancer. A prospective randomized trial. Ann Surg 238:214-220
24. Machado M, Nygren J, Goldman S, Ljungquist O (2005) Functional and physiologic assessment of the colonic reservoir or side-to-end anastomosis after low anterior resection for rectal cancer: a two-year follow-up. Dis Colon Rectum 48:29-36
25. Jiang J-K, Yang S-H, Lin J-K (2005) Transabdominal anastomosis after low anterior resection: a prospective, randomized, controlled trial comparing long-term results between side-to-end anastomosis and colonic J-pouch. Dis Col Rectum 48:2100-2110
26. Ulrich AB, Seiler CM, Z'Graggen K et al (2008) Early results from a randomized clinical trial of colon J-pouch versus transverse coloplasty pouch after low anterior resection for rectal cancer. Br J Surgery 95: 1257-1263
27. Matsuoka H, Masaki T, Kobayashi T et al (2010) Comparison of functional and clinical outcomes: colonic J-pouch vs coloplasty in patients with low rectal cancer. Hepato-gastroenterology 57:70-72
28. Tsunoda H, Kamiyama G, Narita K et al (2009) Prospective randomized trial for determination of optimum size of side limb in low anterior resection with side-to-end anastomosis for rectal carcinoma. Dis Colon Rectum 52:1572-1576
29. Brisinda G, Vanella S, Cadeddu F et al (2009) End-to-end vs End-to-side stapled anastomosis after anterior resection for rectal cancer. J Surg Oncol 99:75-79
30. Bozio G, Mabrut J-Y, Baulieux J (2008) Anastomose colo-anale «différéè», après exérèse totale du mèsorectum par laparoscopie, pour cancer du rectum. J chir 145:262-265
31. Siddiqui MRS, Sajid MS, Woods WGA (2010) A meta-analysis comparing side-to-end with colonic J-pouch formation after anterior resection for rectal cancer. Tech Coloproctol 14:113-123
32. Remzi FH, Gazzaz GE, Kiran RP et al (2009) Outcomes following Turnbull-Cutait abdominoperineal pull-through compared with coloanal anastomosis. Br J Surg 96:424-429

33. Brown CJ, Fenech D, McLeod RS (2008) Reconstructive techniques after rectal resection for rectal cancer. The Cochrane Database of Systematic Reviews 16(2):CD006040
34. Martling AL, Holm T, Rutqvist LE (2000) Effect of a surgical training programme on outcome of rectal cancer in the Country of Stockholm. Stockholm Colorectal Cancer Study Group, Basingstoke Bowel Cancer Research Project. Lancet 356:93-96
35. Rullier E, Laurent C, Bretagnol F et al (2005) Sphincter-saving resection for all rectal carcinomas: the end of the 2-cm distal rule. Ann Surg 241:465-469
36. Pocard M, Sideris L, Zenasni F et al (2007) Functional results and quality of life for patients with very low rectal cancer undergoing coloanal anastomosis or perineal colostomy with colonic muscular graft. Eur J Surg Oncol 33:459-462
37. Portier G, Bonhomme N, Platonoff I, Lazorthes F (2005) Use of Malone antegrade continence enema in patients with perineal colostomy after rectal resection. Dis Colon Rectum 48:499-503
38. Farroni N, Van den Bosch A, Haustermamns K et al (2007) Perineal colostomy with appendicostomy as an alternative for an abdominal colostomy: symptoms, functional status, quality of life, and perceived health. Dis Colon Rectum 50:817-824
39. Gamagami RA, Chiotasso P, Lazorthes F (1999) Continent perineal colostomy after abdominoperineal resection: out come after 63cases. Dis Colon Rectum 42:626-630
40. Kirzin S, Lazorthes F, Nouaille de Gorce H et al (2010) Benefits of perineal colostomy on perineal morbidity after abdominoperineal resection. Dis Colon Rectum 53:1265-1271
41. Abercrombie JE, Williams NS (1995) Total anorectal reconstruction. Br J Surg 82:438-442
42. Schmidt E (1982) The continent colostomy. World J Surg 6:805-809
43. Federov VD, Odaryuk TS, Shelygin YA, Tsarkov PV, Frolov SA (1989) Method of creation of a smooth-muscle cuff at the site of the perineal colostomy after extirpation of the rectum. Dis Colon Rectum 32:562-566
44. Damon H, Guye O, Seigneurin A (2006) Prevalence of anal incontinence in adults and impact on quality-of-life. Gastroenterol Clin Biol 30:7-43
45. Faucheron JL, Hannoun L, Thome C, Parc R (1994) Is fecal continence improved by nonstimulated gracilis muscle transposition? Dis Colon Rectum 37:979-983
46. Christiansen J, Ronholt-Hansen C, Rasmussen O (1995) Bilateral gluteus maximus transposition for anal incontinence. Br J Surg 82:1645-1647
47. Williams NS, Patel J, George BD et al (1991) Development o fan electrically stimulated neoanal sphincter. Lancet 2:1166-1169
48. Baeten CG, Geerdes BP, Adang EM et al (1995) Anal dynamic graciloplsty in the treatment of intractable fecal incontinence. N Engl J Med 332:1600-1605
49. Cavina E, Seccia M, Banti BP, Zocco G (1998) Anorectal reconstruction after abdominoperineal resection: experience with double-wrap graciloplasty supported by low-frequency electrostimulation. Dis Colon Rectum 41:1010-1016
50. Cavina E (1996) Outcome of ristorative perineal graciloplasty with simultaneous excision of the anus and rectum for cancer: a ten-year experience with 81 patients. Dis Colon Rectum 39:182-190
51. Rullier E, Zerbib F, Laurent C et al (2000) Morbidity and functional out come after double dynamic graciloplasty for anorectal reconstruction. Br J Surg 87:909-913
52. Mander BJ, Abercrombie JF, Georg BD, Williams NS (1996) The electrically stimulated neosphincter incorporated as part of total anorectal reconstruction after abdominoperineal excision of the rectum. Ann Surg 224:702-711
53. Rosen HR, Novi G, Zoech G et al (1998) Restoration of anal sphincter function by single stage dynamic graciloplasty with a modified (split-spling) technique. Am J Surg 175:187-193
54. Ho KS, Seow-Chen F (2005) Dynamic graciloplasty for total anorectal reconstruction after abdominoperineal resection for rectal tumor. Int J Colorectal Dis 20:38-41
55. Korsgen S, Keighley MR (1995) Stimulated gracilis neosphincter – not as good as previously thought: report of 4 cases. Dis Colon Rectum 38:1331-1333
56. Romano G, La Torre F, Cutini G et al (2003) Total anorectal reconstruction with the artificial bowel sphincter: report of eight cases. A quality-of life assessment. Dis Colon Rectum 46:730-734

57. Marchal F, Doucet C, Lechaux D et al (2005) Secondary Implantation of an artificial sphincter after abdominoperineal resection and pseudocontinent perineal colostomy for rectal cancer. Gastroenterol Clin Biol 29:425-428
58. Lehur PA, De Kerviler B, Maurel J et al (1997) Constipation morbide de l'adulte: intérets de l'irrigation colique antérograde. Gastroenterol Clin Biol 21:A120
59. Hill J, Scoott S, Maclennan I (1994) Anterograde enemas for the treatment of severe idiopathic constipation. Br J Surg 81:1490-1491
60. Hughes SF, Williams NS (1995) Continent colonic conduit for the treatment of faecal incontinence associated with disordered evacuation. Br J Surg 82:1318-1320
61. Malone PS, Ransley PG, Liely EM (1990) Preliminary report: the anterograde continence enema. Lancet 336:1217-1217
62. Penninckx F, D'Hoore A, Vanden Bosch A (2005) Perineal colostomy with antegrade continence edema as an alternative after abdominoperineal resection for low rectal cancer. Ann Chir 130:327-330
63. Abbes Orabi N, Vanwymersch T, Paterson M (2011) Total perineal reconstruction after abdominoperineal excision for rectal cancer: long-term results of dynamic graciloplasty with Malone appendicostomy. Colorectal Disease 13:406-413

Diverting Stoma

10

Silvia Palmisano, Piera Leon, Simonetta Masaro,
Mattia Trevisan and Nicolò de Manzini

10.1 The Role of Diverting Stoma

The role of a protective stoma is to divert the flow of the feces externally, thus protecting a low colorectal anastomosis which is potentially at risk.

The impact of the stoma on the incidence of anastomotic leakage and related leak mortality is still the object of much debate in literature.

In deciding whether to create a derivative stoma or not, the surgeon must consider that most unprotected patients who develop an anastomotic leakage will require further urgent surgery to create such a stoma, which in 25% of cases will become permanent. However, in the absence of complications, the closure of a temporary stoma is performed in 87.7% of cases [1].

The first studies aimed at clarifying the role of diverting stomas that appeared in literature were carried out on small samples of patients and thus did not reach any definite conclusions [2, 3]. In 2002, a prospective multicenter observational study conducted by the "Colon/Rectum Carcinoma" Working Group (CRCWG) demonstrated that risk of anastomotic leakage requiring surgical reoperation was significantly small thanks to the creation of a protective stoma. The logistic regression analysis performed in this study confirmed that a protective stoma was the strongest and most independent factor in avoiding an anastomotic leakage requiring reoperation (p=0.001) [1].

More recently, in 2007, Matthiessen et al. [4] carried out a randomized multicenter clinical trial on a sample of 234 patients, demonstrating for the first time that the presence of a derivative stoma not only mitigated the disastrous effects of an anastomotic leakage, but also reduced the percentage of

S. Palmisano (✉)
Department of Medicine, Surgery and Health Sciences, General Surgery Unit,
Cattinara University Hospital,
Trieste, Italy
e-mail: silvia.palmisano@aots.sanita.fvg.it

N. de Manzini (ed.), *Rectal Cancer,*
Updates in Surgery
DOI: 10.1007/978-88-470-2670-4_10,

risk of a leak developing. In the past, other authors had reached the same conclusion, but with nonrandomized retrospective multicenter studies [5]. A subsequent meta-analysis of randomized and nonrandomized studies has unequivocally confirmed that a protective stoma significantly reduces both the percentage of leakage and the percentage of reoperations [6].

At the moment, little is known about the effects of a stoma on anorectal function. In 2011, using a questionnaire, a multicenter controlled clinical trial by Lindgren et al. [7] assessed anorectal function in patients undergoing anterior resection of the rectum with and without protective stoma. The questionnaire focused on analysing different parameters: frequency and any difficulties in evacuation, the use of laxatives, incontinence or defecatory urgency, and the impact of the stoma on daily life. Moreover, patients without stoma were asked if they would prefer the creation of a stoma to reduce the impact of changes in anorectal functions, where present. The conclusion of this study was that after one year the presence of a diverting stoma did not cause significant alterations of the anorectal function, and that in any case all the patients preferred reduced anorectal function rather than the creation of a stoma.

10.2 Loop Ileostomy (LI) vs. Loop Colostomy (LC)

The benefits of a stoma in reducing the percentage of anastomotic leakage and in improving the postoperative recovery of patients developing an anastomotic dehiscence must be compared to the percentage of morbidity of the stoma itself and to the mortality related to its closure, which involves a further surgical operation requiring a second hospital admission. A percentage of morbidity up to 36.5% and of mortality up to 1.4% correlated to the closure of the ostomy [1, 8, 9] has been estimated. Furthermore, it has been calculated that the hospital stay of patients with protective stoma is longer than that of patients without stoma, with a consequent increase in health costs. This longer stay is probably due to the time necessary for the patient to get used to managing the stoma [4].

In literature there is no preference as regards the type of protective stoma. According to Law et al. [10] and Gooszen et al. [11], LC gives better results than LI. In particular, according to these authors, the closure of the LI is associated with a greater risk of anastomotic dehiscence and small bowel obstruction and with a mortality rate of 0.5%.

Edwards et al. [12], on the other hand, have pointed out a number of contraindications to LC: a higher rate of parastomal hernias and prolapse, and a greater incidence of post operational hernias, probably connected to an increase in bacterial contamination at the moment of closure. These results were confirmed in a study by Rullier, which demonstrated a percentage of complications connected to the stoma of 35% for LC and 19% for LI, as well as a higher percentage of complications after closure of LC (34%) compared to LI (12%) [13].

More recently, two meta-analyses analysed 5 randomized clinical trials by comparing the efficacy and safety of LC and LI: both only found a smaller and nonsignificant percentage of prolapse associated to LI without, however, demonstrating any real advantage of one technique over the other [14, 15].

In their review of 3 randomized clinical studies and 4 cohort studies, Tilney et al. [16] demonstrated a preference of LI over LC correlated to lower rates of wall infection, global complications, and incisional hernias.

The most recent meta-analysis on the subject was performed by Rondelli et al. [17]; though it analyses a large amount of data and parameters, the study does not definitively show the superiority of one treatment over another, requiring the publication of further controlled clinical trials with a greater number of patients.

A new technique recently introduced to protect distal colorectal anastomosis is Ghost Ileostomy (GI) [18]. The advantage of this technique is that it is only undertaken when there is clinical evidence of anastomotic leakage. There are 2 types: Ghost ileostomy without parietal split, and Ghost ileostomy with parietal split. In both cases the next to last ileal loop is prepared in correspondence to the right iliac fossa and freed from any adherences. In the procedure without parietal split, a Prolene stitch is passed through the mesenteric edge of the ileal loop and exteriorized at the cutaneous skin surface with a Reverdin needle. In the technique with wall incision, a McBurney incision is made, and a pediatric Robinson catheter, which was previously made to pass through the meso of the second to last ileal loop, is exteriorized through this incision. In both cases the ileal loop is suspended under the fascia ready to be exteriorized in the event of anastomotic leakage. In the wall incision technique, the ileostomy may even be created in local anesthesia. If, on the other hand, the anastomosis heals without complications, the Prolene thread and the pediatric Robinson catheter are cut and the intestinal loop is abandoned in the abdomen. The advantage of GI is that the stoma is only opened if an anastomotic leak develops, thus reducing useless stoma, hospitalization for closing the stoma, and health care costs. Furthermore, if the GI has to be opened, stoma-related mortality and morbidity can be likened to that of a classic stoma.

A limitation of this procedure could be the risk of extended fecal contamination of the leakage due to the delayed opening of the stoma. Furthermore, the number of patients undergoing this innovative procedure is extremely small.

To conclude, in literature ileostomy is the operation of choice for elective colorectal surgery to protect the anastomosis, reduce the incidence of leakage, and mitigate undesirable effects; colostomy on the other hand is preferred in emergency operations or reoperations.

10.3 Closing the Stoma

Most derivative stomas are subsequently closed, but in some cases they are transformed into permanent stomas. There may be many reasons for non-closure: refusal by the patient, postoperative complications, clinical conditions of nonoperability, tumor progression, anastomotic stricture, and alteration of continence [19, 20]. It has been estimated that intestinal continuity is not restored in 19.2% of cases [5].

In contrast, in most cases when there are no clinical signs referable to a colorectal leakage, patients with a derivative stoma are recommended for a closing operation. The absence of symptoms or clinical signs of anastomotic leakage is not, however, proof of healing, so that the colorectal anastomosis must be studied before the operation to check its integrity.

In literature there is no unanimous consensus on the type of examination recommended to test the suture, though historically, the examination of choice is the transanal water-soluble contrast enema (WCE). Some authors, including Lim et al. [21], have drawn up a radiological classification of anastomotic leakage and have identified some predictive characteristics of healing or persistence.

Other studies in literature, on the other hand, propose alternative clinical and instrumental examinations to WCE: digital rectal examination and rectosigmoidoscopy [22, 23]. Kaladay et al. [22] proposed a digital rectal examination 4-6 weeks after rectum resection, and a rectoscopy for patients who showed no clinical signs of anastomotic leakage. In the absence of pathological confirmation, closure of the ostomy was programmed two months later without any radiological study of the anastomosis.

In our opinion the best examination for studying the anastomosis is WCE, which should be performed just two weeks after rectal resection. In the event of radiological leakage, another two serial WCEs should be planned at intervals of a month to compare the radiological images. If the radiological images of a leak persisting in clinically asymptomatic patients are stable, we advise closing the ileostomy [24].

Another widely debated matter in literature concerns the most appropriate moment to close the stoma. The closing operation is not usually performed less than 8-12 weeks after the anastomosis has healed. This period should be long enough for the complete reacquisition of the patient's functions after the colorectal operation, for the intraoperative adhesions to become less tenacious, and for the edema of the stoma to resolve. Perez et al. [25] determined a precise cutoff time of around 8.5 weeks after rectal resection , before which there is a significant increase of postoperative complications. Our recently conducted study encourages us to believe that a protective ileostomy can be closed early, about 2-3 weeks after its creation, if the anastomosis has completely healed. We also suggest closing the stoma even when there is persistent radiological leakage, as long as the serial radiological images of WCE are stable in time and show certain features: a short fistula with a blind ending which empties spontaneously into the rectum, and the absence of clinical signs or symptoms of inflammation or generalized sepsis. Indeed, in the follow-up phase, no patient has shown any clinical complication or any readmission to hospital because of complications related to stoma closure [24].

Early stoma closure was also proposed by Bakx et al. [26] in a pilot study. This analysed 27 patients, 18 of whom underwent closure of the stoma during the same hospital stay as that of their rectal operation. The patients who did not show any complications after rectal resection had WCE approximately 7-8 days after the initial operation. In the absence of radiological leakage, the patients were prepared for the stoma closure operation during the same stay, which was, on average, 11 days after the creation of the stoma. The mean follow-up period was 29 weeks, and during this period no complications occurred.

Early closure of the ileostomy was also recommended in other studies, including that of Jordi-Galais et al. [27], with results in line with those reported in Bakx's study. In both cases the sample studied was small, while large randomized studies would be necessary to reach definite conclusions.

Finally, some studies have assessed the development of complications connected to stoma closure in relation to adjuvant treatment. Thalheimer et al. [28] demonstrated that the lowest percentage of complications correlated to stoma closure occurred in the group of patients who underwent the closure operation before the beginning of adjuvant chemo- and/or radiotherapy (12.5%). At the end of the adjuvant therapy, on the other hand, the percentage of complications was 21.2%, while if the stoma was closed during the adjuvant therapy, the percentage of complications rose to 42.9%. A limitation of this study was, however, the very small number of patients in each group.

10.4 Conclusions

A protective stoma reduces both the incidence of anastomotic leakage and the percentage of re-operations. It also allows a conservative treatment of the leak and reduces negative side effects.

There is no unanimous consensus in literature on the type of stoma to perform. The most frequent complication associated to the closing of an LI is small bowel obstruction; those of LC are parastomal hernias, prolapse, and incisional hernias. However, in terms of complications, neither technique is at present better than the other in a statistically significant manner. The trend is to perform an LI in elective operations and an LC in emergency operations or re-operations. Ghost Ileostomy represents an alternative, but its use is not sufficiently widespread to offer significant data.

Historically, the optimal closing time varied from 8 to12 weeks after colorectal resection. Any shorter period than this meant a greater probability of complications. However, in literature various studies on the early closure of the stoma are being compared, with promising results. Our opinion is that the examination of choice for studying the anastomosis is WCE, and we propose early stoma closure even in the presence of a radiological anastomotic leakage, as long as it has a short linear track with a blind ending which spontaneously empties into the rectum, and if there are no clinical signs or symptoms of inflammation or generalized sepsis.

Finally, in agreement with some studies, stoma closure should be programmed before any adjuvant therapy to minimize the risk of complications.

References

1. Gastinger I, Marusch F, Steinert R et al (2005) Working Group Colon/Rectum Carcinoma. Protective defunctioning stoma in low anterior resection for rectal carcinoma. Br J Surg 92:1137-1142
2. Graffner H, Fredlund P, Olsson SA, Oscarson J (1983) Protective colostomy in low anterior resection of the rectum using the EEA stapling instrument: a randomized study. Dis Colon Rectum 26:87-90
3. Pakkastie TE, Ovaska JT, Pekkala ES et al (1997) A randomised study of colostomies in low colorectal anastomoses. Eur J Surg 163:929-933
4. Matthiessen P, Hallbŏŏk O, Rutegård J et al (2007) Defunctioning stoma reduces symptomatic anastomotic leakage after low anterior resection of the rectum for cancer. A randomized multicenter trial. Ann Surg 246:207-214
5. Peeters KC, Tollenaar RA, Marijnen CA et al (2005) Dutch Colorectal Cancer Group. Risk factors for anastomotic failure after total mesorectal excision of rectal cancer. Br J Surg 92:211-216
6. Tan WS, Tang CL, Shi L et al (2009) Meta-analysis of defunctioning stomas in low anterior resection for rectal cancer. Br J Surg 96:462-472
7. Lingren R, Hallbŏŏk O, Rutegård J et al (2011) Does a defunctioning stoma affect anorectal function after low rectal resection? Results of a randomized multicenter trial. Dis Colon Rectum 54:747-752
8. Machado M, Hallbook O, Goldman S (2002) Defunctioning stoma in low anterior resection with colonic pouch for rectal cancer: a comparison between two hospitals with a different policy. Dis Colon Rectum 45:940-905
9. Kaiser AM, Israelit S, Klaristenfeld D et al (2008) Morbidity of ostomy takedown. J Gastrointest Surg 12:437-441
10. Law WL, Chu KW, Choi HL et al (2002) Randomized clinical trial comparing loop ileostomy and loop transverse colostomy for faecal diversion following total mesorectal excision. Br J Surg 89:704-708
11. Gooszen AW, Geelkerken RH, Hermans J et al (1998) Temporary decompression after colorectal surgery: randomized comparison of loop ileostomy and loop colostomy. Br J Surg 85:76-79
12. Edwards DP, Leppington-Clarke A, Sexton R et al (2001) Stoma-related complications are more frequent after transverse colostomy than loop ileostomy: a prospective randomized clinical trial. Br J Surg 88:360-363
13. Rullier E, Le Toux N, Laurent C et al (2001) Loop ileostomy versus loop colostomy for defunctioning low anastomoses during rectal cancer surgery. World J Surg 25: 274-277
14. Lertsithichai P, Rattanapichart P (2004) Temporary ileostomy versus temporary colostomy: a meta-analysis of complications. Asian J Surg 27:202-210
15. Guenaga KF, Lustosa SA, Saad SS et al (2007) Ileostomy or colostomy for temporary decompression of colorectal anastomosis. Cochrane Database Syst Rev (1):CD004647
16. Tilney HS, Sains PS, Lovegrove RE et al (2007) Comparison of outcome following ileostomy versus colostomy for defunctioning colorectal anastomoses. World J Surg 3:1142-1151
17. Rondelli F, Reboldi P, Rulli A et al (2009) Loop ileostomy versus loop colostomy for fecal diversion after colorectal or coloanal anastomosis: a meta-analysis. Int J Colorectal Dis 24:479-488
18. Cerroni M, Cirocchi R, Morelli U et al (2011) Ghost ileostomy with or without abdominal parietal split. World J Surg Oncol 9:92-96

19. den Dulk M, Smit M, Peeters KC et al (2007) A multivariate analysis of limiting factors for stoma reversal in patients with rectal cancer entered into the total mesorectal excision (TME) trial: a retrospective study. Lancet Oncol 8:297-303
20. Bailey CM, Wheeler JM, Birks M, Farouk R (2003) The incidence and causes of permanent stoma after anterior resection. Colorectal Dis 5:331-334
21. Lim M, Akhtar S, Sasapu K et al (2006) Clinical and subclinical leaks after low colorectal anastomosis: a clinical and radiological study. Dis Colon Rectum 49:1611-1619
22. Kalady MF, Mantyh CR, Petrofski J, Ludwig KA (2008) Routine contrast imaging of low pelvic anastomosis prior to closure of defunctioning ileostomy: is it necessary? J Gastrointest Surg 12:1227-1231
23. Cowan T, Hill AG (2005) Ileostomy closure without contrast study is safe in selected patients. ANZ J Surg 75:218-219
24. Palmisano S, Piccinni G, Casagranda B et al (2011) The Reversal of a Protective Stoma Is Feasible Before the Complete Healing of a Colorectal Anastomotic Leak. The American Surgeon 77:1619-1623
25. Perez RO, Habr-Gama A, Seid VE et al (2006) Loop ileostomy morbidity: timing of closure matters. Dis Colon Rectum 49:1539-1545
26. Bakx R, Busch ORC, van Geldere D (2003) Feasibility of early closure of loop ileostomies: a pilot study. Dis Colon Rectum 46:1680-1684
27. Jordi-Galais P, Turrin N, Tresallet C et al (2003) Early closure of temporary stoma of the small bowel. Gastroenterol Clin Biol 27:697-699
28. Thalheimer A, Bueter M, Kortuem M et al (2006) Morbidity of temporary loop ileostomy in patients with colorectal cancer. Dis Colon Rectum 49:1011-1017

Intraoperative Accidents

11

Marco Kosuta, Davide Cosola and Nicolò de Manzini

11.1 Introduction

In spite of standardization and improvements in technique, colorectal surgery remains subject to an intraoperative accident rate that has undergone a slight increase with the advent of laparoscopy [1]. This fact can be correlated to the technical limitations of laparoscopic access, which are its two-dimensional imaging and the loss of tactile sensation [1]. The most updated studies report a global incidence of intraoperative accidents of 10-13% [2, 3]; for rectal surgery this incidence is significantly higher than for colonic surgery (13% vs. 7%) [3]. The most frequent intraoperative complications are hemorrhage, lesions to the bowel, spleen, urethra and bladder, as well as technical difficulties during anastomosis. The risk of technical difficulties during mini-invasive operations for colorectal cancer is higher for surgeons in the learning phase, a phase that is often longer for laparoscopy than for the same procedures carried out in laparotomy; the learning curve for laparoscopic rectal surgery seems to be about 35 operations [4-6]. In analyzing the learning curve of a junior surgeon, the most significant data are the complication rate, the length of the hospital stay and the incidence of re-hospitalization, and not the conversion rate and the length of the operation; indeed, if the operating time does not go down as the experience of the surgeon increases, this often reflects the fact that the more complex individual cases are generally performed by expert surgeons [7].

In our opinion, however, the term "learning curve" should be banned and replaced with the term "tutorage curve", meaning the number of operations, or

M. Kosuta (✉)
Department of Medicine, Surgery and Health Sciences, General Surgery Unit,
Cattinara University Hospital,
Trieste, Italy
e-mail: kosuta1@libero.it

N. de Manzini (ed.), *Rectal Cancer*,
Updates in Surgery
DOI: 10.1007/978-88-470-2670-4_11, © Springer-Verlag Italia 2013

stages of them, during which, to maintain the same quality, a surgeon needs a tutor.

If intraoperative accidents cannot be solved laparoscopically, they may lead to the conversion of the procedure into laparotomy. Colorectal surgery has a higher conversion rate than other laparoscopic operations; this fact is correlated to factors connected to the patient, the illness, the complexity of the case, and the experience of the surgical team [8].

As far as laparoscopic colorectal surgery is concerned, the following statistically significant risk factors have been identified connected with the incidence of intraoperative accidents which resulted in a need for conversion [9]:

- Obesity
- Males
- Low rectum
- Narrow pelvis

In literature the conversion rate is somewhat variable. In the most recent randomized trials, the conversion rate is between 14 and 20% [10], and is higher in rectal surgery than in colon surgery (18.7% rectum vs. 9.5% colon) [11]. This figure can be explained by the intrinsic difficulty of operating in the pelvic cavity.

It is also necessary to consider the impact that an intraoperative accident with subsequent conversion may have on the postoperative course. Patients undergoing conversion to laparotomy due to an intraoperative difficulty have been shown to have a postoperative course more often than not complicated by wound infections, by a delayed resumption of feeding, by a high need for transfusions, and by a statistically higher mortality rate at 30 days [3, 12, 13].

There follows an analysis of the different intraoperative complications broken down into:

- Difficulties during access to the abdominal cavity
- Spleen lesions
- Vascular lesions
- Lesions to the urinary tract
- Creating the anastomosis (Table 11.1)

11.2 Access to the Peritoneal Cavity and Induction of the Pneumoperitoneum

This section only discusses laparoscopic operations, although laparotomic access is not exempt from the possibility of accidents. The methods adopted to induce pneumoperitoneum are either open or closed, with each of these techniques having a minimum percentage possibility of complications. Late diagnosis of these complications may lead to an increase in global mortality. In literature the complications are broken down into:

Table 11.1 Reasons for conversion. In rectal cancer most conversions are due to pelvic difficulties (last 2 columns)

	Conversion Rate	Reasons for conversion					
Author (year)	(%)	Adhesions	Poor views/obesity/bowel distension	Bleeding	Ureteric injury	Narrow pelvis/ inaccessibility of tumors	Tumor fixity/ bulky tumor
Chan (2008) [14]	8.7%	34.1%	6.4%	9.8%	-	9.8%	26.9%
CLASICC (2005) [3]	29%	-	26%	-	-	20%	41%
Gonzales (2005) [15]	23%	-	58%	7%	-	-	-
Tekkis (2005) [5]	10%	37.6%	16%	11.2%	-	-	9.6%
de Manzini (2011) [41]	13.68%	27.03%	17.56%	9.46%	1.35%	-	31.08%
		Technical difficulties / intraoperative complications				Pelvic difficulties	

- Major (0.18%) [16]:
  - visceral lesions
  - vascular lesions
  - lesions of parenchymatous organs
- Minor
  - extraperitoneal insufflations
  - subcutaneous emphysema

There is currently no consensus on the optimal procedure for gaining access to the peritoneal cavity in the obese and nonobese population [17, 18].

The open techniques basically consist of open and semi-open laparoscopy, while the closed ones include Veress needle insertion and gasless direct trocar insertion, or DTI. The main causes of technical difficulty and thus of intraoperative accidents during induction of pneumoperitoneum are: marked obesity, due to the thickness of the adipose tissue, which complicates the procedure and the presence of prior abdominal surgical operations with consequent peritoneal adherences. The open technique (or Hasson technique) is extremely safe in normal-weight patients, because it allows the first trocar to be inserted into the abdomen under direct visual control. For this reason it is the technique preferred by many surgeons; in our experience, almost all colorectal laparoscopic operations used this technique without any particular difficulties. However, a complication incidence for this technique of more than 0.2% is described, with a rate of 0.06% of intestinal lesions [19]. In patients affected by significant obesity, this technique is not easy to perform; indeed, isolation and suspension of the muscle layer in a thick wall is difficult to execute. The Hasson technique also requires suture of the muscular layer to prevent the onset of postlaparotomic hernia on trocar access; this procedure, performed through a small cutaneous incision, has been shown to be complex in the presence of abundant subcutaneous tissue [20].

The so-called closed techniques, mainly involving DTI and Veress needle insertion, are in contrast with the Hasson technique. Induction of pneumoperitoneum by means of insertion is easier to perform in obese patients, avoiding the limitations of open laparoscopy for these patients; it is fairly quick to perform and also avoids CO_2 leakage. For this reason it is preferred by many surgeons, even for normal-weight patients. The use of the Veress needle may cause greater complications in 0.06-1.3% of cases (0.6% lesions of parenchymatous organs; 0.3% visceral/vascular lesions; 0.3% other lesions), and minor complications in 5.9% (3.4% subcutaneous emphysema; 2.5% extraperitoneal insufflations) [21, 22]. Major intraoperative complications can be reduced by respecting a few technical details: insertion in the left hypochondriac in the event of umbilical hernia or suspected adherences in the mesogaster; minimum movement of the needle while inserting; using insufflation pressure lower than 10mmHg to indicate the correct positioning of the device; needle insertion angle of 45° in nonobese patients and 90° in obese ones.

The gasless DTI technique has recently been described as an alternative to the methods described above, although it was initially restricted to gynecological procedures. The DTI technique, compared to Veress needle insertion in normal-weight patients, did not show significant differences in terms of visceral and vascular lesions, air embolism or mortality [21], although few surgeons use it and it does not seem to be recommended at all as a standard technique.

No matter which technique is used to access the abdomen, in most cases intestinal or vesical lesions can be cleared up by direct suture in laparoscopy, and only rarely and for extremely widespread lesions is it necessary to perform conversion with resection of the intestinal tract affected. While vascular lesions are somewhat rare, they are serious, and often require rapid conversion into laparotomy and surgical repair after a temporary hemostasis has been performed.

To sum up, we can say that the choice of technique to access the abdominal cavity and to create pneumoperitoneum are not determined by the incidence of intraoperative complications, which can be serious, though rare. It is of fundamental importance that the intraoperative accident is promptly diagnosed and treated, also in laparoscopy, with a surgical gesture which is often of modest technical difficulty. A small visceral or vascular lesion not recognized during the operation will certainly require re-operation, and often a major laparotomy.

11.3 Spleen Lesions

Lesions of the spleen during laparoscopic rectal surgery are extremely rare, though underestimated due to the lack of literature on the topic. The occurrence rate of this event is lower than 1% [23]. Iatrogenic lesion of the spleen generally occurs during the left coloparietal and coloepiploic detachment; the cause is commonly excessive traction on the colon or on the epiploon. The consequences of damage to the spleen during laparoscopic rectal surgery are an increase in hematic leakage, an extension of hospital stay, an increase in incidence of infections, and postoperative mortality at 30 days. Most (34%) spleen lesions are to the lower part, and in most cases consist of a simple rupture of the capsule (Grade 1-3 of the OIS Spleen Injury Grading Scale); spleen rupture occurs only in a small percentage of cases (Grade 4-5) (4%) [23]. Lesions to the upper part, the posterior parts, and spleen rupture always require splenectomy (100%) [23].

Lesions to the spleen can be reduced if the best possible exposure is obtained, if the anatomic structures are not subjected to excessive traction, and by performing an adequate dissection of the spleen ligaments and any adherences between the spleen and adjoining structures. Many authors also recommend an approach to splenic flexure starting from the posterolateral side and moving towards the medial side, with the intent of reducing the risk of lesions.

Preservation of the spleen in these situations is preferable and is technically feasible in around 25% of cases [23]. Techniques devised to preserve the organ are based on electrocauterization and splenorrhaphy, and can make use of material like oxidised cellulose hemostatic gauze, animal collagen gauze, and fibrogenous and human thrombin-soaked sponges [24] .

In about 7 % of cases, spleen lesions are still not recognized during the operation, and require reoperation and emergency splenectomy [25].

Splenectomy following an intraoperative lesion of the spleen is also considered a negative prognostic factor as regards the oncological outcome of these patients, who show a cancer-specific survival rate at five years dropping with statistical significance from 70 to 47% [25].

11.4 Vascular Lesions

Lesions to abdominal or pelvic vessels in surgery for rectal cancer mainly occur in patients undergoing reoperation where exposure is difficult (obese patients and those with a narrow pelvis) or those undergoing preoperative radiotherapy [26]. Widespread arteriopathy may also make the vessels more susceptible to lesions, especially where there are important bifurcations (origin of the IMA, origin of the RSA); the formation of atheromatous plaques here is characteristic, for hemodynamic reasons.

It is not easy to find articles in literature that report the specific incidence of vascular lesions in rectal cancer surgery; a recent study reports a value of venous lesions close to 1% in patients undergoing gastroenterological and colorectal surgery for malign tumors [27].

In surgical operations for rectal cancer, the procedures involving the highest risk of vascular lesions are isolation and section of the lower mesenteric vessels, after tying; incision of the pelvic peritoneum anteriorly to the ilium vessels; and detachment of the fascia recti from the Waldeyer's fascia, below which there are the presacral veins which, if cut, retract inside the foramen, making hemostasis requiring wax or hemostatic staples a complicated process.

Lesions to smaller size vessels are easy to control with ultrasonic or radiofrequency scalpel or with bipolar forceps, which moreover seem to limit hematic leakage during the operation better than monopolar instruments [28-30].

Whatever vessel is damaged, the repair must be immediate, considering the negative effects on patient outcome: major hematic loss and blood transfusions [31].

Repairs can be made using a direct suture (or termino-terminal anastomosis in the event of complete section) with nonabsorbable monofilament, ligature, metal clips or, in rarer cases, reconstruction with patches (basically in the event of lesions to the iliac vessels).

If there are major vascular lesions during the laparoscopic approach, the strategy does not change. If the lesion and the surgeon's experience should permit, it is preferable to avoid conversion, but if this should be impossible, the change to the open technique must be made once the source of the bleeding is found and when the hemorrhage has been controlled, with hemostasis by compression. In three cases in our experience the lesion of the lower mesenteric artery at the origin was controlled in laparoscopy, in two with conversion after temporary hemostasis. It is interesting to note how in two cases this lesion was caused by the sharp edge of the hemostatic clips.

11.5 Lesions to the Urinary Tract

Iatrogenic lesions of the urinary tract complicate from 1 to 15% of operations involving the pelvis and the retroperitoneum [32, 33]. They mainly affect the ureter and to a lesser extent the bladder and urethra.

Lesions can be prevented by the experience of the surgeon and the systematic intraoperative recognition/protection of the structures (see the chapter on Surgical Technique) [34]. On the other hand, to the unfavorable conditions already described for vascular lesions we must add some anatomic anomalies: ureteral duplication (1/125), retrocaval ureter, "horseshoe" kidney, and pelvic kidney (1/400). These may increase the difficulty in recognising and respecting the structures, especially if not found in the preoperative stage [35] .

The use of ureteral stents has long been recommended as a possible aid to the surgeon, whereas more recently the use of endoluminal stents has been introduced for the same purpose. The advantages of this procedure are undoubtedly an easier and quicker (up to 45 minutes less) determination of the ureters, against a slight increase in the operating time (approximately 12 minutes) required for positioning the stent, and no incidence of complications regarding the procedure (if we exclude the appearance of hematuria, which is spontaneously resolved). However, it should be said that the positioning of a stent is not always possible and means an increase in costs [32, 36, 37]. In our experience, the use of stents is justified in particular cases (reoperations, extremely voluminous tumors, previous episodes of acute diverticulitis), and should be indicated by the surgeon on the basis of his/her experience and of the clinical and anatomical conditions of the patient. It is not actually a very widely used method.

In rectal surgery, the urinary tract most at risk is the ureter, which may undergo lesions at three key moments: during detachment of Toldt's fascia, at the moment of incision of the pelvic peritoneum anteriorly to the iliac vessels, and during dissection of the lateral ligaments of the rectum.

A lesion at the level of the ureter may occur by section, ligature, devascularization or transmitted thermal damage. In the first two cases, recognition of the lesion should ideally be immediate or in any case before the end of the operation, maybe with the aid of intraoperative pyelography or injection, either intravenous or, through the vesical catheter, of methylene blue. Section caused by an ultrasonic or radiofrequency scalpel does not usually result in urine leakage in the operating field, which may make intraoperative recognition of the lesion difficult. Correction must also be immediate (if it is a laparoscopic operation, the surgeon must decide whether to opt for conversion or not), by means of termino-terminal spatulated anastomosis with interrupted stitches in reabsorbable thread, on the guide of a ureteral stent, which is kept in place after the operation and removed after 4-6 weeks. In the event of accidental ligature of the bowels, the obstruction should simply be removed and, again, a stent should be positioned [33].

Devascularization is a much rarer event, considering the many collateral blood supply networks of the ureter; it is usually associated to a postirradiation state, and is generally revealed with the onset of late stenosis.

Thermal damage has been reduced but not eliminated by the advent of ultrasonic or bipolar scalpels [30, 38]. Lesions from thermal damage, if recognized intraoperatively, can be treated by positioning a stent which prevents stenosis and which should be monitored and replaced until complete healing. If the lesion is revealed by a stenosis or a fistula after the operation, it will be necessary to reconstruct the bowel: the type of operation will depend on the extent of the lesion (ureteral end to end anastomosis , or ureteral reimplantation in bladder associated or not with nephropexy, Boari flap or Psoas hitch): a description of these can be seen in a treatise of urological surgical techniques.

Vesical lesions [39] are generally caused, in rectal surgery, by insertion of the hypogastric trocar, and are treated by suturing the peritoneal breach and with extended vesical catheterization.

Urethral lesions, on the other hand, are almost exclusively related to the perineal phases of abdominoperineal amputation in males, and can be easily avoided by ensuring that the ureteral bulb (easily recognized, also thanks to the presence of the vesical catheter) is not included at the moment of incision.

11.6 Creating the Anastomosis

The surgical stage of creating the anastomosis may be complicated by two opposing types of accident: immediate dehiscence of the rectal stump after sectioning the bowels with a mechanical stapler, and a positive hydropneumatic test result once the anastomosis has been created.

The first case is generally due to a wrong assessment of the thickness of the rectal wall; factors contributing to an increased thickness of the rectal wall are typically neoadjuvant radiotherapy or an incorrect preparation of the bowel up to the *muscolaris propria*. The error may be recognized immediately or at the moment the circular stapler is inserted; in the first case the repair is made with a continuous suture, while in the second case a purse-string stitch can be created around the staple, helping the exposure with the movement of the stapler itself.

Table 11.2 Schematic flow chart in the case of intraoperative anastomotic dehiscence, following anastomotic level and leak severity

	Severity of leak	
Anastomotic level	Light	Severe
Intraperitoneal	Hand sewn suture	ReDo colorectal anastomosis
Extraperitoneal	Hand sewn transanal suture/no suture	ReDo coloanal anastomosis

If the hydropneumatic test (see the chapter on Surgical Technique) is positive, in this case too the anastomotic defect must be sutured, and the hydropneumatic test repeated. In such a situation, the use of vital staining (methylene blue), which would risk confusing the structure rather than identifying the defect, is not recommended. The lower the anastomosis, the more difficult or even impossible it becomes to perform the laparoscopic suture. This may lead, in the event of a complete dehiscence of the anastomosis, to rectal resection and creation of a coloanal anastomosis with all the annexed functional consequences.

It has recently been proposed to perform the hydropneumatic test in reverse (water in the rectum and gas in the abdomen) and to visualise very low anastomoses transanally, with the assistance of devices used for proctological surgery; this method also makes it possible to correct a partial dehiscence by means of direct suture [40]. Finally, a small very low anastomosis dehiscence may be treated with a derivative stomy alone (Table 11.2).

The decision in favor of conversion must be made by the surgeon on the basis of his/her experience and the clinical and anatomic conditions of the patient, whereas anastomosis must be considered a high risk procedure and must be protected with ileostomy or colostomy.

11.7 Conclusions

Intraoperative accidents in rectal surgery may be connected to laparoscopic access, whereas whatever access method used, splenic and especially vascular lesions are the most frequent and dangerous. Ureteral lesions can be prevented using a standardized surgical technique, but above all must be recognised during the course of the operation. Anastomotic imperfections must be subjected to an adequate control algorithm.

References

1. D'Annibale A, Morpurgo E, Fiscon V et al (2004) Robotic and laparoscopic surgery for treatment of colorectal diseases. Dis Colon Rectum 47:2162-2168
2. Tarik S, Arman K, Sanket S et al (2011) Laparoscopic Colorectal Surgery Is Associated With a Higher Intraoperative Complication Rate Than Open Surgery. Ann Surg 253:35-43

3. Guillou PJ, Quirke P, Thorpe H et al, for the MRC CLASICC trial group (2005) Short-term endpoints of conventional versus laparoscopicassisted surgery in patients with colorectal cancer (MRC CLASICC trial): multicentre, randomised controlled trial. Lancet 365:1718-1726
4. Jamali FR, Soweid AM, Dimassi H et al (2008) Evaluating the degree of difficulty of laparoscopic colorectal surgery. Arch Surg 143:762-767
5. Tekkis PP, Senagore AJ, Delaney CP, Fazio VW (2005) Evaluation of the learning curve in laparoscopic colorectal surgery: comparison of right-sided and left-sided resections. Ann Surg 242:83-91
6. Li GX, Yan HT, Yu J et al (2006) Learning curve of laparoscopic resection for rectal cancer. Nan Fang Yi Ke Da Xue Xue Bao 26:535-538
7. Kirchhoff P, Clavien PA, Hahnloser D (2010) Complications in colorectal surgery: risk factors and preventive strategies. Patient Safety in Surgery 4:5
8. Shawki S, Bashankaev B, Denoya P et al (2009) What is the definition of "conversion" in laparoscopic colorectal surgery? Surg Endosc 23:2321-2326
9. Thorpe H, Jayne DG, Guillou PJ et al (2008) Patient factors influencing conversion from laparoscopically assisted to open surgery for colorectal cancer. Br J Surg 95:199-205
10. Chan ACY, Poon JTC, Fan JKM et al (2008) Impact of conversion on the long-term outcome in laparoscopic resection of colorectal cancer. Surg Endosc 22:2625-2630
11. Tan PY, Stephens JH, Rieger NA, Hewett PJ (2008) Laparoscopically assisted colectomy: a study of risk factors and predictors of open conversion. Surg Endosc 22:1708-1714
12. Li JCM, Lee JFY, Ng SSM et al (2010) Conversion in laparoscopic-assisted colectomy for right colon cancer: risk factors and clinical outcomes. Int J Colorectal Dis 25:983-988
13. Yang C, Wexner SD, Safar B et al (2009) Conversion in laparoscopic surgery: does intraoperative complication influence outcome? Surg Endosc 23:2454-2458
14. Chan ACY, Poon JTC, Fan JKM et al (2008) Impact of conversion on the long-term outcome in laparoscopic resection of colorectal cancer. Surg Endosc 22:2625-2630
15. Gonzalez R, Smith CD, Mason E et al (2006) Consequences of conversion in laparoscopic colorectal surgery. Dis Colon Rectum 49:197-204
16. Ahmad G, Duffy JMN, Phillips K et al (2008) Laparoscopic Entry Techniques. Cochrane Database of Systematic Reviews Issue 2. Art. No.: CD006583. DOI: 10.1002/14651858
17. Merlin TL, Hiller JE, Maddern GJ et al (2003) Systematic review of the safety and effectiveness of methods used to establish pneumoperitoneum in laparoscopic surgery. Br J Surg 90:668-679
18. Molloy D, Kaloo PD, Cooper M, Nguyen TV (2002) Laparoscopic entry: a literature review and analysis of techniques and complications of primary port entry. Aust N Z J Obstet Gynaecol 42:246-255
19. Jacobson MT, Osias J, Bizhang R et al (2002) The direct trocar technique: an alternative approach to abdominal entry for laparoscopy. JSLS 6:169-174
20. Madan AK, Menachery S (2006) Safety and Efficacy of Initial Trocar Placement in Morbidly Obese Patients. Arch Surg. 141:300-303
21. Agresta F, DeSimone P, Ciardo LF et al (2004) Direct trocar insertion versus Veress needle in nonobese patients undergoing laparoscopic procedures. Surgical Endoscopy 18:1778–81
22. Schäfer M, Lauper M, Krähenbühl L (2001) Trocar and Veress needle injuries during laparoscopy. Surg Endosc 15:275-80
23. Merchea A, Dozois EJ, Wang JK, Larson DW (2012) Anatomic Mechanisms for Splenic Injury During Colorectal Surgery. Clin Anat 25:212-217
24. Holubar SD, Wang JK, Wolff BG et al (2009) Splenic Salvage After Intraoperative Splenic Injury During Colectomy. Arch Surg 144:1040-1045
25. Wakeman CJ, Dobbs BR, Frizelle FA et al (2008) The impact of splenectomy on outcome after resection for colorectal cancer: a multicenter, nested, paired cohort study. Dis Col Rect 51:213-217
26. Kirchhoff P, Clavien PA, Hahnloser D (2010) Complications in colorectal surgery: risk factors and preventive strategies. Patient Saf Surg 4:5

27. Oktar GL (2007) Iatrogenic major venous injuries incurred during cancer surgery. Surg Today 37:366-369
28. Hubner M, Demartines N, Muller S (2008) Prospective randomized study of monopolar scissors, bipolar vessel sealer and ultrasonic shears in laparoscopic colorectal surgery. Br J Surg 95:1098-1104
29. Hubner M, Hahnloser D, Hetzer F et al (2007) A prospective randomizedcomparison of two instruments for dissection and vessel sealing in laparoscopic colorectal surgery. Surg Endosc 21:592-594
30. Noble EJ et al (2011) Experimental comparison of mesenteric vessel sealing thermal damage between one bipolar and two ultrasonic shears devices Br J Surg 98:797-800
31. Kirchhoff P, Dincler S, Buchmann P (2008) A multivariate analysis of potential risk factors for intra- and postoperative complications in 1316 elective laparoscopic colorectal procedures. Ann Surg 248:259-265
32. Redan A, McCarus SD (2009) Protect the Ureters Jay. JSLS 13:139-141
33. Delacroix SE Jr, Winters JC (2010) Urinary Tract Injures: Recognition and Management Clin Colon Rectal Surg 23:104-129
34. Larach SW, Patankar SK, Ferrara A (1997) Complications of laparoscopic colorectal surgery. Analysis and comparison of early vs. latter experience. Dis Colon Rectum 40:592-596
35. Fröber R (2007) Surgical anatomy of the ureter. BJU Int 100:949-965
36. Chahin F, Dwivedi A, Paramesh A et al (2002) The implications of lighted ureteral stenting in laparoscopic colectomy. J Soc Laparoendosc Surg 6:49-52
37. Nam YS, Wexner SD (2002) Clinical Value of Prophylactic Ureteral Stent Indwelling During Laparoscopic Colorectal Surgery. J Korean Med Sci 17:633-635
38. Emam T, Cuschieri A (2003) How safe is high-power ultrasonic dissection. Ann Surg 237:186-191
39. van Goor H (2007) Consequences and complications of peritoneal adhesions. Colorectal Dis 9:25-34
40. Crafa F (2011) Anastomoses très basses avec CAD. III Journées francophones de Chirurgie Colorectale sous Coelioscopie, Napoli 23-25/11/2011
41. de Manzini N (2012) Unpublished data

Postoperative Complications 12

Michela Giuricin, Greta Giacomel, Alessandra Lucchetta
and Nicolò de Manzini

12.1 Introduction

In this chapter we classify the complications of rectal surgery into early and late, according to the moment when they usually occur. For all the complications we have indicated the therapy, in some cases more than one, recently reported in literature. Late complications connected to lesions of the nerve plexus are treated in the dedicated chapter.

12.2 Early Complications

12.2.1 Anastomotic Hemorrhages

Postoperative hemorrhage is a complication that may occur early or late. In 85% of cases it occurs during the first postoperative day, whereas it is very rarely found beyond the 10th day after the operation [1]. This chapter deals with postoperative anastomotic hemorrhages; intraoperative hemorrhages have already been discussed in a previous chapter.

The incidence of hemorrhage after mechanical anastomosis varies from 0 to 2.5% up to 6.5% [2, 3]. In a review published in the 2001 Cochrane Database, Lustosa et al. found an incidence of anastomotic hemorrhages after colorectal resection of 5%, observing how in mechanical anastomosis the hemorrhage occurs in 5.4% of cases, against 3.4% after handsewn anastomosis [4].

M. Giuricin (✉)
Department of Medicine, Surgery and Health Sciences, General Surgery Unit,
Cattinara University Hospital,
Trieste, Italy
e-mail: michelagiuricin@libero.it

N. de Manzini (ed.), *Rectal Cancer*,
Updates in Surgery
DOI: 10.1007/978-88-470-2670-4_12,

In the most recent study, performed by Ishihara in 2008, which involved 73 patients subjected to colorectal surgery with mechanical anastomosis, postoperative bleeding was observed in 9.6% of cases. In this study an intraoperative colonoscopy was routinely performed in all patients to reveal the source of the bleeding and perform immediate hemostasis [5].

Anastomotic hemorrhage is in most cases self-limiting and is clinically manifested with rectal bleeding [3]. In these cases a conservative approach is now the best choice, and may consist not only in clinical observation alone, but also in blood transfusion and rectal packing.

In the rare cases in which the hemorrhage is not self-limiting (Cirocco reports a severe bleeding incidence in 1% of cases), the therapy must be surgical [3]. In these cases the first choice approach is endoscopic: through colonoscopy, the hemostasis can be controlled by positioning metallic clips, injecting submucosal adrenalin, or using both methods. However, electrocoagulation and sclerotherapy with submucosal adrenaline can give rise to complications like the development of necrosis of the suture line and the possible formation of an anastomotic leak [6], although the occurrence rate is very low. In a single study of 73 patients, colonoscopy was used intraoperatively, ensuring surgical hemostasis under endoscopic control [5]. In the rare cases refractory to endoscopic therapy, another safe choice for the patient is endovascular therapy: selective angiography with embolization or vasopressin injection [7]. However, in literature, it is well-known that this choice is affected by complications like infarction, intestinal ischemia or hemorrhagic infarction [8].

In low anastomoses it is also possible to perform transanal surgery with the various methods of low rectal access now available (operating proctoscope, devices for stapled hemorrhoidectomy, TEM).

12.2.2 Conclusions

- Postoperative hemorrhage is a complication that may occur early or late. It occurs in 85% of cases during postoperative day one, whereas it is very rarely found beyond the 10th day after the operation.
- The incidence of hemorrhage after mechanical anastomosis varies from 0 to 2.5% up to 6.5%.
- Anastomotic hemorrhage is in most cases self-limiting and is clinically manifested through rectal bleeding. In the rare cases in which it is not self-limiting, the therapy must be surgical. The first choice approach is endoscopic. In the rare cases refractory to endoscopic therapy, another choice is the use of endovascular therapy: selective angiography.
- In low anastomoses it is possible to perform transanal surgery: operating proctoscope, devices for stapled hemorrhoidectomy, TEM.

12.3 Anastomotic Leakage

Anastomotic leakage is major cause of morbidity and mortality after anterior resection (AR). A 2010 Cochrane study showed that anastomotic dehiscence determined a perioperative mortality of between 2 and 24% [9]. In literature, however, there is currently no unequivocal definition of anastomotic dehiscence [10]. In some studies, in fact, only leaks detected clinically and radiologically are considered [11-13], whereas in other studies only dehiscences necessitating early re-operation are examined [14, 15]. Rahbari's recent review of 59 articles on anastomotic dehiscence after colorectal surgery defines the anastomotic leak as a communication between the intra- and extra-luminal compartments caused by a defect of integrity of the intestinal wall at the level of the colorectal or coloanal anastomosis [10]. These different definitions explain the variability in the incidence of leaks in literature, from 3% to 39% [10, 16, 17].

However, it is well known that clinical leaks are less frequent than radiological ones, as can be seen from Buchs' prospective study (2008), where he reports that the percentage of clinical leaks is only from 3 to 6 % of the total [13].

Of the risk factors for the development of anastomotic leaks, male sex (already identified by Rullier in his 1998 study) is now confirmed as an independent factor by a Cochrane review of 2010 [18, 9]. Obesity, diabetes mellitus and the level of anastomosis are also confirmed as contributing factors by Hotta et al.'s 2011 literature review [19].

Neoadjuvant radiotherapy was, however, identified as an independent risk factor by Matthiessen in 2004, by Jones in 2007 and by Harris in 2010 [20-22]. In Zhu's study of 2010, on the other hand, tumor diameter exceeding 3 cm and the stage of the illness at the moment of surgery were indicated as risk factors [23]. Of the predisposing factors, it has now been ascertained that those connected to the surgical technique and to the operator must always be included: the surgeon's experience, type of anastomosis, and number of mechanical stapler charges used [24, 25].

In 1997 Vignali indicated that a distance of less than 7 centimetres from the anal verge entailed a high risk of dehiscence in rectal anastomosis [26]. This fact now becomes important if we consider that the distal safety margin from the tumor was reduced to 5 and now 2 centimetres, allowing increasingly lower resections-anastomoses [11, 20, 27].

If an anastomotic leak should occur, it is vital for it to be recognized immediately with an assessment of the general and local conditions of the patient [27]. Hemodynamically stable patients without signs or symptoms of sepsis can be treated with conservative therapy: medical therapy, maintaining drain, or US-guided drainage of any collections.

Re-operation is indicated when conservative therapy fails and if there is sepsis: this involves intestinal resection and reanastomosis, delay in the closure of a protective stoma or creation of a new protective stoma, resection without anastomosis (Hartmann resection, temporary or definitive), use of occlusive agents like fibrin glue [28]. In our experience, two cases of a leak with abscess of a significant size were rapidly resolved by surgical positioning of pararectal drainage.

A stoma can be used routinely in low resections or as a salvage method in association with drainage of postoperative collections. However, in literature, the real effect of the routine use of the stoma during AR is still widely debated [29] and is discussed in chapter 10.

Some authors report a reduction of leakage and re-operation in patients undergoing protective ileostomy [10, 30, 31].

On the other hand, others, like Matthiessen in 2004 and Wong in 2005, do not consider the stoma a crucial factor in reducing leaks [11, 32]. However, in his restrospective study of 2006, Magdalena acknowledges the protective stoma's capacity for reducing clinical leaks by increasing the subclinic rate, although it does not really modify the total percentage [33]. Nevertheless, the creation of an extremely distal and particularly difficult anastomosis under tension, or an excessive dissection which determines insufficient blood supply are factors aiding the formation of leaks in AR [23].

The use of abdominal drainage is still extremely controversial. It used to be thought that abdominal drainage would reduce the formation of leaks by reducing postoperative residual fluid collection [34]; however, in a meta-analysis of 4 randomized trials in 1999, Urbach demonstrated that the use of abdominal drainage is not associated with any reduction in the development of leaks [35]. More recent studies have shown that the routine use of pelvic drainage does not reduce the incidence of anastomotic leaks, because all the abdominal fluids cannot be evacuated by drainage [36].

The last few years have seen the development of new therapeutic approaches to anastomotic leaks. Interest has focused in particular onthe different endoscopic techniques permitting debridement of the abscess cavity and closure of the fistulous tract (positioning stents, injecting fibrin glue, use of vacuum therapy). Chopra's retrospective study assesses the short- and long-term results of different endoscopic techniques in 13 patients with anastomotic leaks: millimetric leaks were treated with fibrin glue, whereas leaks of less than 2 cm and located in the middle-high rectum were treated by positioning stents [37].

Literature studies confirm that endoluminal self-expanding plastic stents (SEPS) and metal stents have the potential to promptly close the leak [38]. However, their limited use and the complications connected to them should always be considered: migration of the stent and patient discomfort, especially if used in the lower rectum [39], and last but not least, the possible risk of intestinal perforation [40]. Larger leaks may be treated with vacuum therapy: in the last few years a number of studies have examined the treatment of colorectal leaks associated to paranastomotic abscesses with the placement of a sponge and an associated continuous pressure device [41, 42].

Since the end of the 1990s it has been demonstrated that vacuum therapy facilitates healing of external wounds, thanks to its continuous mechanism of increasing microcirculation, decontamination, and enhanced granulation tissue formation [43]. These same principles are, therefore, also applied to healing the leak and their associated abscessual cavity.

As well as demonstrating the good results of these innovative techniques, Chopra's study also reports the long-term complications . These include anastomotic stenosis and blind leaks [37]. Further studies in literature envisage the use of new endoscopic devices like specially created endoclips for the treatment of colorectal leaks [44]. It must, however, be emphasized that further prospective studies are necessary to validate the new endoscopic methods in the treatment of leaks after colorectal surgery.

12.3.1 Conclusions

- In literature there is currently no unequivocal definition of anastomotic dehiscence,; this explains the variability of incidence, which ranges from 3% to 39%.
- If an anastomotic fistula should occur, it is vital for it to be recognized immediately, with an assessment of the general and local conditions of the patient. Conservative therapy is the first approach, but if the patient's general condition deteriorates, or if the initial therapy fails, re-operation is generally required.
- The routine use of a stoma during AR is still widely debated; the use of abdominal drainage is also still extremely controversial.
- New therapeutic approaches include endoscopic techniques with positioning stents, or injecting fibrin glue, or use of Vacuum therapy. However, a long-term complications have also been reported with these innovative techniques.

12.4 Infections of the Surgical Site

Surgical site infection (SSI) holds third place amongst the most common hospital-acquired infections, and colorectal surgery is the elective procedure with greatest incidence of SSI.

The National Nosocomial Infection Surveillance System (NNIS) of the Centers for Disease Control and Prevention (CDC) classifies SSI into incisional (surface and deep) and infections of organs/cavities connected to the surgical operation [45, 46]. It has now been ascertained that this complication doubles the risk of postoperative mortality, increases the risk of readmission by approximately 5 times and extends hospitalization from 5 to 20 days, with a consequent increase in the associated costs.

The frequency of SSI is different according to whether the operation site is the colon or the rectum. In rectal surgery more stomas are performed, preoperative radiotherapy is frequent, and the anastomoses are closer to the anal verge; all these procedures prolong the operating time and the risk of bacterial contamination, and contribute to making the rectum the site of the highest SSI [47]. The application of prevention systems has partially reduced the incidence of wound infections, which have a rate reported in literature between 3 and 38% [45-47].

A recent prospective multicenter observational study carried out by Serra-Aracil on 611 patients reports an incidence of SSI after surgery exclusively for rectal neoplasia of 27.6%, with a predominance of incisional infections and with more than a fifth of SSIs diagnosed after discharge. Of the many possible risk factors for incisional SSI, the only one found to have significance in the univariate analysis is the ASA score ($p=0.03$), whereas for the infections of organs/cavities, independent predictive factors in multivariate analysis are hyperglycemia at 48 hours ($p=0.047$) and a temperature of less than 36°C at the beginning of the operation ($p=0.005$). It also seems that the incidence of this complication varies according to the size of the hospital, with an increase in hospitals with fewer than 250 beds, but it appears that this applies basically to colon surgery. In another study Konishi points to preoperative radiotherapy, cortisol treatment, and the creation of a stoma as predictive factors for incisional SSI [47].

A retrospective study in 2011 by Ho et al. on 650 patients who underwent either colon or rectal surgery for tumor or MICI reports that incisional SSIs (12.6%) are multifactorial, and does not identify any statistically significant risk factor. Infections of organs/cavities (9.9%) are, in the same study, correlated to the level of preoperative albumin, to a history of pelvic radiotherapy, to operations classified as contaminated, and to postoperative hyperglycemia ($p<0.059$) [46].

In Poon et al.'s prospective study published in 2009 and carried out on 1,011 patients subjected to colorectal resection, the incisional SSI (4.8%) risk factors were anastomotic dehiscence ($p>0.01$), perioperative transfusions ($p=0.047$) and an open resection ($p=0.037$); whereas organ/cavity (1.8%) infections seem to be correlated only to dehiscence of the anastomosis ($p<0.01$) [45].

As historical studies by Miles and Burke show, suitable antibiotic prophylaxis may reduce the rate of infection of the surgical site. A meta-analysis of the 2009 Cochrane review demonstrates that the risk of SSI decreases with any antibiotic prophylaxis regimen compared to placebo alone. The retrospective study carried out by Ho et al. on 650 patients, quoted above, indicated that the most frequently used antibiotic regimen is cefazolin+metronidazole, and that the patients who receive nonstandardized treatment regimens have an increased risk of SSI, whereas the standardized ones (cefoxitin, cefazolin+metronidazole, metronidazole+fluoroquinolone) all have comparable efficacy. The administration of the antibiotics should ideally be timed to allow their concentration in the tissue at the moment of the incision, but there is disagreement about the optimum moment of administration, either 30 or 60 minutes before incision. However, the current guidelines establish that they must be given within one hour prior to incision [48].

In 2007 the Surgical Care Improvement Project (SCIP) drew up a series of measures designed to reduce the SSI incidence rate. These envisage the following: timing of administration of prophylactic antibiotics (PAs) within 1 hour of incision; using approved PA regimens; and discontinuing PA within 24 hours [49]. Euglycemia should be maintained, with well-controlled morning blood glucose concentrations on the first two post-operative days, especially in cardiac surgery patients; hair at the surgical site should be removed with clippers or by depilatory methods, not with a blade; urinary catheters are to be removed within the first two post-operative days; and normothermia should be maintained peri-operatively [50].

The objective was to reduce SSI incidence by 25% before 2010 by implementing these measures; studies assessing these results mainly agree in asserting that the adoption of these measures has led to a reduction of SSI, but that further improvement is necessary. In particular, Edmiston et al. suggests that in the future it would be better not to focus on reducing single risk factors for SSI, but rather on various measures like: preadmission antiseptic showering, state-of-the-art skin antisepsis, innovative antimicrobial technology, active staphylococcal surveillance, and pharmacological and physiological considerations only in selected patients [51-54].

12.4.1 Conclusions

- SSI are divided into incisional (surface and deep) infections and infections of organs/cavities associated to the operation.
- Many risk factors have been analysed. The only ones uniformly determined are perioperative hyperglycemia and preoperative temperature, and during the operation infections of organs/cavities, while no risk factor has been shown to be significant for incisional infections.
- The current guidelines (SCIP) focus particularly on antibiotic prophylaxis, the use of standardized regimens and appropriate timing for their administration (within 1 hour prior to incision), but they should be further implemented and adjusted to the individual patient and to the various risk factors.

12.5 Late Complications

12.5.1 Anastomotic Stenosis

Rectal stenosis has been defined as the impossibility of passing a rigid instrument with an external diameter of 19 mm through an anastomosis, although some authors further reduce the circumference, defining stenosis as the inability to pass through the anastomosis using a flexible sigmoidoscope with a diameter of 12.3 mm [55].

The frequency of benign stenosis after colorectal anastomosis ranges from 0 to 30%. No specific cause is reported for this complication, but contributing factors indicated include ischemia, hemorrhage, anastomotic leaks, pelviperitonitis, obesity, and adjuvant radiotherapy; some authors also report the anastomotic technique and the presence of a proximal protective stoma [55-58].

In a prospective study carried out on 179 patients with colorectal anastomosis, Bannura et al. highlighted a proximal stoma, benign disease and male sex as risk factors for the onset of a stenosis. The same study showed that, paradoxically, the risk of stenosis was greater when using circular staplers with a diameter of 31/34 mm and even more so with those of a diameter of 28/29 mm, compared to those of 25 mm routinely used in the hospital [55].

There is also an ongoing debate regarding manual or mechanical anastomosis: which of the two is more frequently associated with stenosis? In their meta-analysis of randomized clinical studies including 1,233 patients, Lustosa SA et coll. did not succeed in demonstrating the superiority of one technique over the other as regards the formation of anastomotic stenosis, data supported by a previous multicenter study by Docherty et al. on 1,161 patients [59, 60].

However, a recent study by Polese et al. highlights the use of mechanical staplers as one the most important risk factors for developing anastomotic stenosis; furthermore, the same study showed that operations for diverticular disease had a higher incidence of anastomotic stenosis than cancer surgery [61].

However, not all stenoses are symptomatic; symptomatic stenoses requiring treatment are only a part of the radiological ones. Literature reports a rate that ranges from 6 to 73 % of anastomotic stenoses requiring some form of treatment, a wide range which shows that each patient has to be assessed individually and on a clinical basis, and not only according to the results of radiological and endoscopic examinations [62, 55, 61]. We must, however, take into consideration the fact that the majority of authors use mechanical suturing in anastomosis on the subperitoneal rectum, and that the hand sewn versus stapled debate is almost always irrelevant for low colorectal anastomoses. Finally, the data on anastomotic stenosis after operations for diverticular disease tell us that the features of the transposed colon wall also have a role in causing the stenoses [63].

The aim of dilating an anastomotic stenosis is to reach a greater circumferential diameter: at least 13 mm according to the standard criteria in literature [57].

Since the beginning of the 1980s, endoscopic dilatation of anastomotic stenosis has been shown to be a more than valid alternative to surgery. Currently the most common endoscopic procedure carried out is pneumatic balloon dilatation: a procedure associated to a low complication rate and with a success rate at 6-24 months from the first procedure of more than 90% [57, 58].

How many dilatations are recommended? The number reported in literature is absolutely variable: up to 7 or even 13 sessions [64].

In our opinion this number of sessions appears excessive; our experience suggests that more than 4 dilatations without any sign of clinical improvement indicates the necessity of a surgical solution, if the general conditions of the patient should permit.

A recent comparative study by Xinopoulus et al. of the use of the classic balloon and metal olive dilators in a group of patients with rectal anastomotic stenosis showed equal efficacy of the two methods, though there are undoubted economic advantages in using the latter instrument rather than the balloon, as it can be used for more than one session [58].

Another alternative to using the balloon alone, proposed by Andicoechea Agorrìa et al., is the association of this treatment with intralesional injections of cortisone, specifically triamcinolone acetonide, a solution already adopted for stenoses in oesophageal surgery or in cases of intestinal stenosis in subjects with Crohn's disease. The study reported only two cases but it seemed interesting to mention it as an alternative [65].

In the event of tight stenosis, some authors, including Mukai et al., suggest using an electrified hook endoscopically for incision of the mucosa and submucosa, followed by pneumatic dilatation. This procedure obviously requires considerable experience on the part of the endoscopist [66]. Transanal stapled resection of the stenotic ring has also been proposed.

In our experience, pneumatic dilatation has often given good results on a clinical level and as far as the quality of life of the patients is concerned. If three sessions of pneumatic dilatation do not give the desired result, we recommend surgery. We have no personal experience of the other alternative indicated above, but we think it worthwhile to provide as complete an overview of the available therapies as possible.

12.5.2 Ischemic Stenosis

A stenosis longer than the height of the anastomosis may be of ischemic origin, connected to excessive traction on the transposed colon and its vessels, which has not caused an acute dehiscence but a chronic ischemia that slowly leads to fibrosis. There is not much data on this in literature, but many authors have sporadic experience of this situation . In our experience we had 2 cases of male patients, slim, smokers, radiated, with low anastomoses protected by stoma, without postoperative leaks or other septic complications, in whom radiological examination showed a stenosis of at least 5 cm, smooth, concentric without recurrence of tumor. The treatment adopted was Redo Surgery, with delayed closure of the stoma (Fig. 12.1).

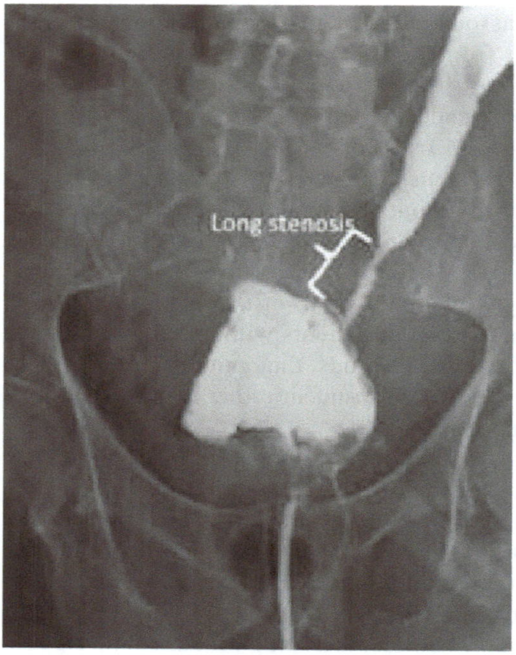

Fig. 12.1 Contrast enema showing a long ischemic stenosis (*bracket*) following an uncomplicated colorectal anastomosis

12.5.3 Conclusions

- The frequency of benign stenosis after colorectal anastomosis ranges from 0 to 30%.
- Literature does not report a specific cause for this type of complication, but contributing factors include ischemia, hemorrhage, anastomotic leaks, pelviperitonitis, obesity, and adjuvant radiotherapy; some authors also report the anastomotic technique, the presence of a proximal protective stoma, and diverticular disease.
- Symptomatic stenoses requiring some kind of therapeutic procedure are only a part of the radiological ones.
- Endoscopic dilatation of anastomotic stenosis has been shown to be a more than valid alternative to surgery.

12.6 Rare Complications

12.6.1 Portomesenteric Thrombosis

Deep venous thrombosis is a very rare but potentially lethal complication after rectal surgery.

Venous thrombosis is generally characterized by a multifactorial etiology [67]. There is a strong family tendency to thrombophilia, with factors that have been recognized for years: factor V Leiden mutation, deficiency of proteins C, S and antithrombin III, etc.

The best-known locoregional predisposing factors which reduce the portal blood flow include abdominal trauma, malign neoplasms, inflammatory abdominal disease, and cirrhosis.

Laparoscopic surgical procedures are, however, of more recent interest [68].

These, including laparoscopic surgery of the rectum, cause an increase in endoabdominal pressure, which consequently determines a reduced portal and mesenteric venous flow [69].

Furthermore, the transperitoneal diffusion of CO_2 causes hypercapnia, which determines an increase of the portal venous pressure and an increase of the mesenteric peripheral resistances, further reducing the venous flow [70].

Another hypothesis is longer maintenance of the Trendelenburg position, which in some experimental studies resulted in major venous stasis. Some cases describe the existence of a thrombus in the stump of the inferior mesenteric vein, left for too long.

However, it can never be excluded that during a surgical operation it is the surgical act itself and the direct lesion of the endothelium which may determine the onset of Virchow's triad.

The clinical manifestation may vary widely, from total absence of symptoms to intestinal ischemia, up to septic shock. In most cases patients exhibit nonspecific abdominal pain (90%) and gastrointestinal symptoms (vomiting, diarrhea, nausea, gastrointestinal bleeding). The abdominal drainage may assume a chylous character [71, 72].

On a laboratory level, it is not rare to find leucocytosis, metabolic acidosis, and an increase in hepatic function assessment [73].

In his 2009 review, James reports a range of symptom appearance from 3 to 42 days, with an average of 14 days [71].

The gold standard for diagnosis is the computed tomography with contrast medium, which reaches a sensitivity of 90% [74, 75] (Fig. 12.2).

The therapy involves immediately beginning anticoagulant treatment, which should last from no less than 6 months up to 12 months. Different studies report partial or total vascular recanalization in 90% of the patients treated with heparin and EBPM [76]. Some other studies with small numbers of patients report the use of endovascular thrombolysis [77, 78], also after positioning a TIPS.

In literature there is a single case of spontaneous resolution after splanchnic venous thrombosis, reported by Davies in 2002 [79].

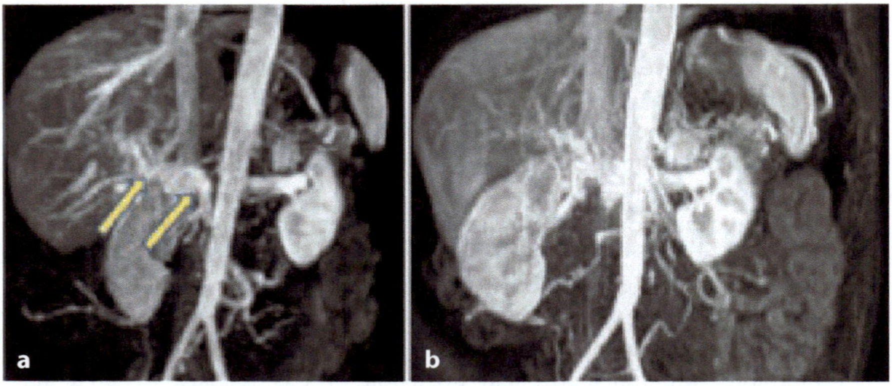

Fig. 12.2 MRI of portal thrombosis following laparoscopic colorectal resection for rectal cancer. **a** At 12° post op day, (*arrows*). **b** Portal vein recanalized at month 6 after anticoagulant therapy

References

1. Martinez-Serrano MA, Parés D, Pera M et al (2009) Management of lower gastrointestinal bleeding after colorectal resection and stapled anastomosis. Tech Coloproctol 13:49-53
2. Hedberg SE, Helmy AH (1984) Experience with gastrointestinal stapling at the Massachussetts General Hospital. Surg Clin North Am 64:511-528
3. Cirocco WC, Golub RW (1995) Endoscopic treatment of postoperative hemorrhage from a stapled colorectal anastomosis. Am Surg 61:460-463
4. Lustosa SA, Matos D, Atallah AN et al (2001) Stapled versus hand-sewn methods for colorectal anastomosis surgery. Cochrane Database Syst Rev CD003144
5. Ishihara S, Watanabe T, Nagawa H et al (2008) Intraoperative Colonoscopy for stapled anastomosis in colorectal surgery. Surg Today 38:1063-1065
6. Perez RO, Sousa AJr, Bresciani C et al (2007) Endoscopic management of postoperative stapled colorectal anastomosis hemorrhage. Tec Coloproctol 11:64-66
7. Weldon DT, Burke SJ, Sun S et al (2008) Interventional management of lower gastrointestinal bleeding. European Radiology 18:857-867
8. Jander HP, Russinovich NA (1980) Transcatheter gelfoam embolization in abdominal, retroperitoneal, and pelvic hemorrhage. Radiology136:337-344
9. Montedori A, Cirocchi R, Farinella E et al (2010) Coverying ileo- or colostomy in anterior resection for rectal carcinoma (Review). Cochrane Database Syst Rev (5):CD006878
10. Rahbari NN, Weitz J, Hohenberger W et al (2010) Definition and grading of anastomotic leakage following anterior resection of the rectum: a proposal by the international study group of rectal cancer 147:339-351
11. Matthiessen P, Hallböök O, Rutegård J et al (2007) Defunctioning stoma reduces symptomatic anastomotic leakage after low anterior resection of the rectum for cancer: a randomized multicenter trial 246:207-214
12. Lipska MA, Bissett IP, Parry BR et al (2006) Anastomotic leakage after lower gastrointestinal anastomosis: men are at a higher risk. ANZ J Surg 76:579-585
13. Buchs NC, Gervaz P, Secic M et al (2008) Incidence, consequences, and risk factors for anastomotic dehiscence after colorectal surgery: a prospective monocentric study. Int J Colorectal Dis 23:265-270
14. Lee WS, Yun SH, Roh YN et al (2008) Risk factors and clinical outcome for anastomotic leakage after total mesorectal excision for rectal cancer. World J Surg 32:1124-1129

15. Ye F, Wang D, Xu X et al (2008) Use of intracolonic bypass secured by a biodegradable anastomotic ring to protect the low rectal anastomosis. Dis Colon Rectum 51:109-115
16. Guillou PJ, Quirke P, Thorpe H et al (2005) Short term endpoints of conventional versus laparoscopic-assisted surgery in patients with colorectal cancer (MRC CLASICC trial): multicentre, randomised controlled trial. Lancet 365:1718-1726
17. Bruce J, Krukowski ZH, Al-Khairy G et al (2001) Systematic review of the definition and measurement of anastomotic leak after gastrointestinal surgery. Br J Surg 88:1157-1168
18. Rullier E, Laurent C, Garrelon JL et al (1998) Risk factors for anastomotic leakage after resection of rectal cancer. Br J Surg 85:355-358
19. Hotta T, Yamaue H (2011) Laparoscopic surgery for rectal cancer : review of published literature 2000-2009. Surg Today 41:1583-1591
20. Matthiessen P, Hallböök O, Andersson M et al (2004) Risk factors for anastomotic leakage after anterior resection of the rectum. Colorectal Dis 6:462-469
21. Jones OM, John SK, Horseman N et al (2007) Low anastomotic leak rate after colorectal surgery: a single-centre study. Colorectal Dis 9:740-744
22. Harris LJ, Phillips BR, Maxwell PJ et al (2010) Outcomes of low anterior resection anastomotic leak after preoperative chemoradiation therapy for rectal cancer. Am Surg 76:747-751
23. Zhu QL, Feng B, Lu AG et al (2010) Laparoscopic low anterior resection for rectal carcinoma: complication and management in 132 consecutive patients. World J Gastroenterol 16:4605-4610
24. Kim JS, Cho SY, Min BS, Kim NK (2009) Risk factors for anastomotic leakage after laparoscopic intracorporeal colorectal anastomosis with a double stapling technique. J Am Coll Surg. 209:694-701
25. Ito M, Sugito M, Kobayashi A et al (2008) Relationship between multiple numbers of stapler firings during rectal division and anastomotic leakage after laparoscopic rectal resection. Int J Colorectal Dis 23:703-707
26. Vignali A, Fazio VW, Lavery IC et al (1997) Factors associated with the occurence of leaks in stapled rectal anastomoses : a review of 1014 patients. J Am Coll Surg 185:105-113
27. Do L, Syed N, Puthawala A et al (2011) Low-lying rectal cancer with anal canal involvement: abdominoperineal or low anterior resection after neoadjuvant chemoradiotherapy. Gastrointest Cancer Res 4:90-95
28. Arumainayagam N, Chadwick M, Roe A (2009) The fate of anastomotic sinuses after total mesorectal excision for rectal cancer. Colorectal Disease 11:288-290
29. Hüser N, Michalski CW, Erkan M et al (2008) Systematic review and meta-analysis of the role of defunctioning stoma in low rectal cancer surgery. Annals of Surgery 248:52-60
30. Marusch F, Koch A, Schmidt U et al (2002) Value of a protective stoma in low anterior resection for rectal cancer. Dis Colon Rectum 45:1164-1171
31. Gastinger I, Marusch F, Steinert R et al (2005) Protective defunctioning stoma in low anterior resection for rectal carcinoma. Br J Surg 92:1137-1142
32. Wong NY, Eu KW (2005) A defunctioning ileostomy does not prevent clinical anastomotic leak after a low anterior resection: a prospective, comparative study. Dis of Col Rect 48:2076-2079
33. Lipska MA, Bissett IP, Parry BR et al (2006) Anastomotic leakage after lower gastrointestinal anastomosis: men are at a higher risk. ANZ J Surg 76:579-585
34. Gingold BS, Jagelman DG (1982) Value of pelvic suction-irrigation in reducing morbidity of low anterior resection of the rectum a ten year experience. Surgery 91:394-398
35. Urbach DR, Kennedy ED, Cohen MM (1999) Colon and rectal anastomoses do not require routine drainage: a systematic review and meta-analysis. Ann Surg 229:174-180
36. Yeh CY, Changchien CR, Wang JY et al (2005) Pelvic drainage and other risk factors for leakage after elective anterior resection in rectal cancer patients: a prospective study of 978 patients. Annals of surg 241:9-13
37. Chopra SS, Mrak K, Hünerbein M (2009) The effect of endoscopic treatment on healthing of anastomotic leaks after anterior resection of rectal cancer. Surgery 145:182-188

38. Scileppi T, Li JJ, Iswara K et al (2005) The use of a Polyflex coated esophageal stent to assist in the closure of a colonic anastomotic leak. Gastrointest Endosc 62:643-645
39. Hünerbein M, Krause M, Moesta KT et al (2005) Palliation of malignant rectal obstruction with self-expanding metal stents. Surgery 137:42-47
40. Trovato C, Fiori G, Ravizza D et al (2006) Delayed colonic perforation after metal stent placement for malignant colorectal obstruction. Endoscopy 38:E96
41. Mees ST, Palmes D, Mennigen R et al (2008) Endo-vacuum assisted closure treatment for rectal anastomotic insufficiency. Dis Colon Rectum 51:404-410
42. Arezzo A, Miegge A, Garbarini A, Morino M (2010) Endoluminal vacuum therapy for anastomotic leaks after rectal surgery. Tech Coloproctol 14:279-281
43. Morykwas MJ, Argenta LC, Shelton-Brown EI et al (1997) Vacuum-assisted closure: a new method for wound control and treatment: animal studies and basic foundation. Ann Plast Surg 38:553-562
44. Parodi A, Manta R, Pedroni A et al (2011) Trattamento di fistole e perforazioni del tratto gastroenterico. Giorn Ital End Dig 34:47-52
45. Poon JT, Law W, Wong IW et al (2009) Impact of laparoscopic colorectal resection on surgical site infection. Ann Surg 249:77-81
46. Ho VP, Stein SL et al (2011) Differing risk factors for incisional and organ/space surgical site infections following abdominal colorectal surgery. Dis Colon Rectum 54:818-825
47. Serra-Aracil X, Garcia-Domingo MI et al (2011) Surgical site infection in elective operations for colorectal cancer after the application of preventive measures. Arch Surg 146:606-612
48. Ho VP, Barie PS (2011) Antibiotic regimen and the timing of prophylaxis are important for reducing surgical site infection after elective abdominal colorectal surgery. Surg Inf 12:255-260
49. Nguyen N, Yegiyants S, Kaloostian C et al (2008) The Surgical Care Improvement project (SCIP) initiative to reduce infection in elective colorectal surgery: which performance measures affect outcome? Am Surg 74:1012-1016
50. Rosenberger LH, Politano AD, Sawyer RG (2011) The surgical care improvement project and prevention of post-operative infection, including surgical site infection. Surg Infect 12:163-168
51. Alexander JW, Solomkin JS, Edwards MJ (2011) Updated recommendations for control of surgical site infections. Ann Surg 253:1082-1093
52. Edmiston CE, Spencer M, Lewis BD (2011) Reducing the risk of surgical site infections: did we really think SCIP was going to lead us to the promised land? Surg Infect 12:169-177
53. Rosenberger LH, Politano AD, Sawyer RG (2011) The surgical care improvement project and prevention of post-operative infection, including surgical site infection. Surg Infect 12:163-168
54. Hawn MT, Vick CC, Richman J et al (2011) Surgical site infection prevention: time to move beyond the surgical care improvement program. Ann Surg 254:494-499
55. Bannura GC, Cumsille MA, Barrera AE et al (2004) Predictive factors of stenosis after stapled colorectal anastomosis: prospective analysis of 179 consecutive patients. World J Surg 28:921-925
56. Curcio G, Spada M, di Francesco F et al (2010) Completely obstructed colorectal anastomosis: a new non-electrosurgical endoscopic approach before balloon dilatation. World J Gastroenterol 16:4751-4714
57. Nguyen-Tang T, Huber O, Gervaz P, Dumonceau JM (2008) Long-term quality of life after endoscopic dilation of strictured colorectal or colocolonic anastomoses. Surg Endosc 22:1660-1666
58. Xinopoulos D, Kypreos D, Bassioukas SP et al (2011) Comparative study of balloon and metal olive dilators for endoscopic management of benign anastomotic rectal strictures: clinical and cost-effectiveness outcomes. Surg Endosc 25:756-763
59. Lustosa SA, Matos D, Atallah AN, Castro AA (2002) Stapled versus handsewn methods for colorectal anastomosis surgery: a systematic review of randomized controlled trials. Sao Paulo Med J 120:132-136

60. Docherty JG, McGregor JR, Akyol AM et al (1995) Comparison of manually constructed and stapled anastomoses in colorectal surgery. West of Scotland and Highland Anastomosis Study Group. Ann Surg 221:176-184
61. Polese L, Vecchiato M, Frigo AC et al (2012) Risk factors for colorectal anastomotic stenoses and their impact on quality of life: what are the lessons to learn? Colorectal Dis 14:e124-e128
62. Marchena Gómez J, Ruiz de la Cuesta E, Gómez Guerra G et al (1997) Anastomotic stricture with the EEA-Stapler after colorectal anastomosis. Rev Esp Enferm Dig 89:835-842
63. Ambrosetti P, Francis K, De Peyer R, Frossard JL (2008) Colorectal anastomotic stenosis after elective laparoscopic sigmoidectomy for diverticular disease: a prospective evaluation of 68 patients. Dis Colon Rectum 51:1345-1349
64. Nguyen-Tang T, Huber O, Gervaz P et al (2008) Long- term quality of life after endoscopc dilatation of strictured colorectal or colocolonic anastomoses. Surg Endosc 22:1660-1666
65. Andicoechea Agorría A, Quintela Baizán I, Del Casar Lizcano JM et al (2011) Combined endoscopic ballon dilation and intralesional corticosteroid treatment of colorectal anastomotic stenosis refractary to dilatation alone. Cir Esp [Epub ahead of print]
66. Mukai M, Kishima K, Iizuka S et al (2009) Endoscopic hook knife cutting before balloon dilatation of a severe anastomotic stricture after rectal cancer resection. Endoscopy 41:e193-e194
67. Wang JT, Zhao HY, Liu YL (2005) Portal vein thrombosis. Hepatobiliary Pancreat Dis Int 4:515-518
68. Abdelrazeq AS, Dwaik MA, Aldoori MI et al (2006) Laparoscopy-associated portal vein thrombosis :description of an envolving clinical syndrome. J Laparoendosc Adv Surg Tech A 16:9-14
69. Ishizaki Y, Bandai Y, Shimomura K et al (1993) Changes in splanchnic blood flow and cardiovascular effects following peritoneal insufflation of carbon dioxide. Surg End 7:420-423
70. Epstein RM, Wheeller Ho, Frumin MJ et al (1961) The effect of hypercapnia on estimeted hepatic blood flow, circulating splanchinic blood volume and hepatic sulfobromophthalein cleaance during general anesthesia in man. J Clin Invest 40:592-598
71. James AW, Rabl C, Westphalen AC et al (2009) Portomesenteric Venous Thrombosis after Laparoscopic Surgery. Arch Surg144 : 520-526
72. Vadalà S, Cinardi N, Li Volti G et al (2008) Portal vein thrombosis following laparoscopic total mesorectal excision: case report. Tech Coloproctol 12:259-261
73. Macpherson A (1984) Portal hypertension doe to extrahepatic portal venous obstruction: a review of 40 cases. J R Coll Surg Edinb 29:4-10
74. Bradbury MS, Kavanagh PV, Bechtold RE et al (2002) Mesenteric venous thrombosis: diagnosis and non invasive imaging. Radiographics 22:527-541
75. Hidajat N, Stobbe H, Griesshaber V et al (2005) Imaging and radiological interventions of portal vein thrombosis. Acta Radiol 46:336-343
76. Condat B, Pessione F, Helene Denninger M et al (2000) Recent portal or mesenteric venous thrombosis: increased recognition and frequent recanalization on anticoagulant therapy. Hepatology 32:466-470
77. Aytekin C, Boyvat F, Kurt A et al (2001) Catheter-directed thrombolysis with transjugular access in portal vein thrombosis secondary to pancreatitis. Eur J Radiol 39:80-82
78. Sze DY, O'Sullivan GJ, Johnson DL et al (2000) Mesenteric and portal venous thrombosis treated by transjugular mechanical thrombolysis. AJR 175:732-734
79. Davies M, Satyadas T, Akle CA (2002) Spontaneous resolution of a superior mesenteric vein thrombosis after laparoscopic Nissen fundoplication. Ann R Coll Surg Engl 84:177-180

Surgical Strategy: Indications 13

Nicolò de Manzini, Piera Leon, Paola Tarchi and Massimo Giacca

13.1 Introduction

Modern improvements in instrumental imaging have led to an increase in our knowledge of the anatomy and natural history of rectal cancer. Surgical techniques have gone through developments aimed at improving radicality while preserving sphincter integrity and pelvic innervations at the highest quality level; on the other hand, the goal of exploring a less invasive approach for early-stage tumors has also been pursued.

Surgical anatomy of the mesorectum and the techniques of complete exeresis have now been completely defined, and the preservation of the sphincter for low rectal tumors remains the main issue; in contrast, the evolution of laparoscopic techniques, the introduction of robotic surgery, the anterior-transanal combined techniques or the transanal isolated approach are more recent fields of application that have extended the range of surgery.

Furthermore, the role of multimodality therapies has been recognized as a worldwide standard, to the extent that the response to neoadjuvant therapy has become a strong decision-making factor in better defining surgical indications and proper timing. To plan the most appropriate therapeutic strategy, we need to focus on the various surgical access options (laparoscopy, laparotomy), and on strategies for very early and locally-advanced tumors, with particular regard to the response of low rectal cancer tumors to neoadjuvant therapy, in which strategy decisions are even more difficult to take and can have major consequences.

N. de Manzini (✉)
Department of Medicine, Surgery and Health Sciences, General Surgery Unit,
Cattinara University Hospital,
Trieste, Italy
e-mail: nicolo.demanzini@aots.sanita.fvg.it

N. de Manzini (ed.), *Rectal Cancer,*
Updates in Surgery
DOI: 10.1007/978-88-470-2670-4_13,

13.2 Surgical Access: Laparotomy, Laparoscopy, Robot, SILS and NOTES

13.2.1 Laparotomy and Laparoscopy

Laparotomy has always been considered the classical surgical approach in colorectal operations, but during the last twenty years laparoscopy has emerged as a mini-invasive alternative, especially for the treatment of colonic cancer. Randomized clinical trials focusing on the technical feasibility and oncological long-term results of laparoscopy have already been officially validated [1-3].

Compared to cancer of the colon, rectal cancer presents greater technical difficulties, linked to pelvic dissection, complete and atraumatic exeresis of the mesorectum, and nerve preservation, but also to the difficulty of low rectal section with mechanical staplers, which initially were not suited to this purpose. All this has been discussed in the previous chapters.

These issues have delayed the routine use of laparoscopy in rectal cancer surgery; this is justifiable, considering that laparoscopic colorectal surgery is still not predominantly widespread in any specific country, but has been developed and standardized only in dedicated high-volume centers [4]. After the publication of the randomized controlled studies on the role of laparoscopy in colon cancer, many studies specifically focusing on its use in rectal cancer appeared in the literature, with the primary goal of proving the validity of laparoscopy in terms of immediate, functional and long-term oncological results. Some of the most significant studies are shown in Table 13.1 [5-11].

The technical difficulty of laparoscopic rectal resection is demonstrated by the high conversion rate (the definition of which is not standardized in literature), although this rate varies according to the type of studies considered (mono- or multicentric) and the period in which they were carried out. The CLASICC [1] study was one of the first multicentric randomized controlled trials (RCT); it clearly showed that over time the conversion rate dropped from 36 to 16%. Reviewing the different series, it is not always possible to identify the real causes of the conversion: sometimes it is due to obesity, other times to the location of the tumor [12], intraoperative accidents [12], and difficult anatomic situations or locally-advanced tumors not seen in the pre-operative imaging (as described in Chapter 11). Some authors assert that conversion leads to an increased risk of postoperative complications [1, 12-14], but this hypothesis is not confirmed in other studies [9, 11]. Distal section of the low rectum in a narrow pelvis is undoubtedly a difficult maneuver, but this is now partially predictable on the basis of preoperative elements like MRI and the patient's gender [15, 16]; on the other hand, it can be improved with experience, new techniques like transanal pull through [17] and the quality of the instruments, as we saw in the chapter on resection techniques.

Complications directly related to colorectal resection are basically the consequence of anastomotic dehiscence, which in all papers has the same inci-

Table 13.1 Immediate results of laparoscopic rectal resection

Author (year)	Study type	Open/lap	Conversion	Mortality open/lap	Morbidity open/lap	Anastomotic dehiscence open/lap
Morino et al. (2005) [5]	NR	93/98	18.4%	2.2/1% NS	23.6/24.4% NS	5.1/13.5% NS
Braga et al. (2007) [6]	R	85/83	7.2%	1.1/1.2% NS	40/28.9% NS	10.6/9.6% NS
CLASICC (2007) [1]	R	128/253	34%	-	14/18% NS	7/8% NS *
Strohlein et al. (2008) [7]	NR	275/114	21.9%	3.3/0% NS	-	15.3/10.1% NS
Laurent et al. (2009) [8]	NR	233/238	15%	2.6/0.8% NS	20.2/22% NS	6.4/5% NS
Park et al. (2009) [9]	NR	374/170	0	0	4.8/5.8% NS#	5.7/5.7% NS
Kang et al. (2010) [10]	R	170/170	2%	0	23.5/21.2% NS	0/2% NS
de Manzini et al. (2012) [11]	NR	52/130	16%§	1.9/1.8% NS	7.7/0.9% p=0,03	5.8/10.1% NS

R, randomized; NR, non-randomized case matched.
* Reports dehiscence of 15% and accrued morbidity and mortality in converted patients.
# Only complications requiring reoperation.
§4/21 conversions with enlarged Pfannenstiel, 10/21 with limited midline, 7/21 midline.

dence in laparotomy or laparoscopy [1-10], except in one controlled study where there is a difference in favor of laparoscopy [18]. Long stenosis of an ischemic nature is a less frequent complication [19], even if it is difficult to assess the exact incidence and prevalence on the basis of surgical access. In contrast, the significant advantage for the abdominal wall is described by almost all the authors in terms of incidence, seriousness and socioeconomic impact of surgical site infections [10, 20, 21, 22] and, for some, also as regards long-term incisional hernia [23]. A wide-ranging French survey concludes that laparoscopy has lower postoperative mortality and that it is an independent factor of better immediate outcome [24].

Laparoscopy has the advantage of leading to better functional results; these are not so evident in the CLASICC study [1], which, however, makes no distinction between colon and rectum. An improvement in the quality of life after rectal cancer resections is, on the other hand, demonstrated in both monocentric [6, 25] and multicentric studies [10], while it cannot be assessed in the two meta-analyses published [20, 26]. If we consider bladder and sexual dysfunctions, the results of a randomized study of 10 years ago were worse for laparoscopy [27], while more recent data are significantly better, despite lower levels of evidence [28-30]. It is important to take into account the fact that preservation of the sexual function is not inevitably constant in males, especially when a combination of surgery and radiotherapy is needed; the patient's sexual function should therefore be one of the items included in preoperative consent.

The short-term oncological results of laparotomy and laparoscopy are basically the same: the three main criteria regarded as a standard of surgical specimen quality are the number of lymph nodes, distal margin and circumferential margin (CRM), basically comparable in all controlled studies. A summary of these data is given in Table 13.2.

Overall long-term survival and disease-free survival are also comparable, while for some authors converted patients have a higher risk of recurrence [1]; in one study [32], the cancer-specific survival rate of converted patients is not different from that of non-converted patients, even though conversion and related complications may affect overall survival. In many series this data is of minor importance, probably due to greater recent attention to preoperative imaging, which has led both to a strict selection of patients and a reasoned choice of conversion. However, authors who found a relation between intraoperative difficulties and long-term prognosis should also be mentioned [33]. In our experience, conversion has no influence on mortality, morbidity or long-term survival. Survival was not affected negatively by laparoscopy in any of the controlled studies published. As for port-site metastasis, observed mainly in the early, pioneering days of laparoscopy, monocentric series [9] and meta-analyses [20, 26] do not currently describe a higher incidence than that historically reported in open surgery [34]. The main results are given in Table 13.3.

In conclusion, laparoscopy has a consolidated role in rectal cancer surgery, with short- and long-term results in line with those of open surgery. It has now

Table 13.2 Immediate oncological results: quality of the specimen

Author (year)	Study type	Open/lap	Lymph nodes	CRM <1mm	Distal margin +	R+
Aziz et al. (2006) [20]	META	-	NS	10.8/9.5% NS	-	-
Zhou et al. (2004) [18]	R	89/82	-	-	0	
CLASICC (2007) [1]	R	128/253	13.5/12 NS	14/16% NS	-	-
Braga et al. (2007) [6]	R	85/83	13.6/12.7 NS	2.3/1.2% NS	0	-
Breukink et al. [26]	META	-	NS	-	NS	-
Strohlein et al. (2008) [7]	NR	275/114	16.9/13.5 p0.001	-	-	10/3% NS
Laurent et al. (2009) [8]	NR	233/238	-	6/7% NS	0.9/2.9%NS	5.2/8% NS
Park et al. (2009) [9]	NR	374/170	18/17 NS	4.1/2.9%NS	NS	-
Kang et al. (2010) [10]	R	170/170	18/17 NS	4.1/5.2% NS	0	
Trastulli et al. (2012) [31]	META	-	NS	NS	NS	-
de Manzini et al. (2012) [11]	NR	52/130	20/21 NS	5.7/1.5% NS	0	0

META, meta-analysis; *R*, randomized; *NR*, non-randomized, case matched.

Table 13.3 Late oncological results

Author (year)	Study type	Open/lap	Port site metastases	Local relapse	Overall survival	Relapse free survival
Aziz et al. (2006) [20]	META	-	NS	10.8/9.5% NS	-	-
CLASICC (2010) [35]	R	128/253	2	8.7/10.8% NS	52.9/60% NS	52.1/53.2% NS §
Braga et al. (2007) [6]	R	85/83	-	2.3/1.2% NS	0	-
Strohlein et al. (2008) [7]	NR	275/114	1*	9.5/6.9%NS	NS#	
Laurent et al. (2009) [8]	NR	233/238	-	5.5/3.9% NS	0.9/2.9%NS	79/82% NS @
Park et al. (2009) [9]	NR	374/170				
de Manzini (2012) [11]	NR	52/130	1*	5.7/1.5% NS	0	- @°

META, meta-analysis; *NS*, non-significant; *R*, randomized; *NR*, non-randomized case matched; § OS for converted patients 49.6% p=0.05; *together with peritoneal carcinomatosis; #in subgroup with deep anterior resection survival was significantly better in laparoscopic group; @no worse OS in converted patients; °significantly better in stage III subgroup.

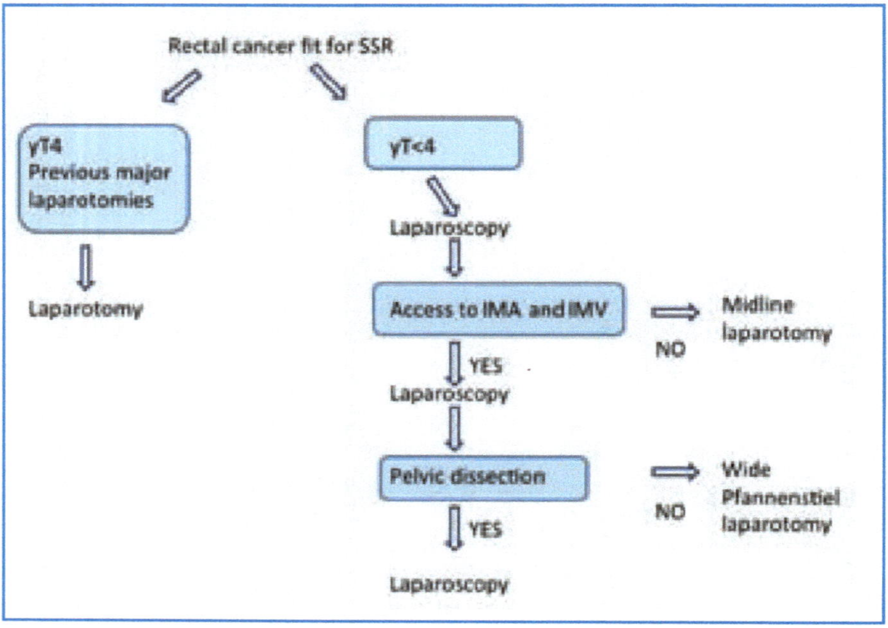

Fig. 13.1 Operating protocol for choosing laparotomy, laparoscopy and kind of conversion

been proven beyond doubt that the oncological results are comparable, even if some details of conversions need to be clarified. T4 tumors are contra-indicated for laparoscopy, due to the high risk of conversion and perforation; however, these are cases which can now be diagnosed preoperatively with MRI. At present, one single study does not, however, report worse results even for T4 tumors [36]. The best oncological results that could have been hoped for from experimental evidence or microscopic observation [37] have not been confirmed in clinical practice, at least until now, and it may be necessary to wait for the results of ongoing trials [38] before getting an answer, although it is objectively difficult today to include patients in these randomized studies. The advantage for the abdominal wall is clear, and consists of less frequent and serious infections, lower rates of incisional hernia, and a saving of the "parietal capital", which allows more specific surgical strategies for advanced tumors to be implemented [39, 40]. An extremely specific preoperative work-up together with the technical standardization and experience of the surgical team contribute to a high level of quality of surgical exeresis, which should no longer be affected by the learning curve [13]. In our opinion this term should be abandoned in favor of a term reflecting the high-quality level of the team, called the *proficiency-gain curve* [41], based on the improving autonomy of surgeons under training. Figure 13.1 illustrates our operating protocol for open and laparoscopic rectal resection, for the choice of the correct parameters for conversion.

13.2.2 Robotic Surgery

The technical and technological limitations of laparoscopy can be summarized as its two-dimensional vision (2-D), limited, 4-degrees-only mobility of the instruments inside the abdomen, a fixed insertion point and possible poor coordination between hand and instrument. The current robotic system allows 3D vision, with the camera integrated into a stable operative platform, magnified vision with zoom, use of instruments with 7 degree freedom of movement, improved ergonomics, and a filter for movements and tremors. These advantages appear to be useful, especially in the event of a narrow pelvis, as has been proved by experience in radical prostatectomies. In monocentric studies, feasibility and short-term results are in line with those of laparoscopic surgery [42-45].

Until now, three meta-analyses have shown robotic surgery to be as good as laparoscopy, the main objection being cost, deemed to be higher (but very few trials report data on costs, and none presents statistically significant differences) [46-48].

All the meta-analyses consider the operating times (longer for robotic surgery, mainly due to the time necessary for the correct positioning of the machine, which has to be changed several times during rectal resection), length of hospitalization, conversion rate, anastomotic dehiscence, and short-term oncological outcome. These results are summarized in Table 13.4.

To conclude, robotic surgery is not inferior to laparoscopic surgery, either oncologically or as regards short-term outcomes. However, there is a lack of prospective randomized trials: the first study is still ongoing, requires 400 patients, and its structure was published only in August 2011 [49].

In an era when costs and cost-benefit ratio have an increased bearing on public health, the main limit to the development of robotic surgery seems to be economic. Furthermore, the current development of 3D-cameras for laparoscopic surgery might in future make it possible to reduce the first disadvantage of conventional laparoscopy we mentioned above.

13.2.3 Single-port (SILS) and NOTES

Laparoscopic rectal cancer surgery through a single port has been described very little in case reports and today can be considered merely experimental, although it is feasible in the studies published [50, 51]. Furthermore, the possibility that this technique, like others, is industry-driven should be considered, and we must try to understand if its technical complexity is offset by real clinical advantages.

On the other hand, much has been said about Natural Orifice Transluminal Endoscopic Surgery (NOTES) in abdominal surgery, although there are few studies on colorectal carcinoma [52] and almost none focusing specifically on rectal carcinomas [53]. This concept was initially applied to transanal extrac-

Table 13.4 Meta-analysis for robotic rectal surgery

Author (year)	N. studies	N. patients	Technique	Operating time	Length of stay	Conversion rate	Leak rate	Oncological outcome
Leong et al. (2011) [46]	9	434	5hybrid 3 full robot 1 mixt	Ns in 3 R>L in 2	NS	Favors R	NS	N° nodes: NS DM:NS CRM:NS
Lin et al. (2011) [47]	8	661	-	NS	NS	Favors R	NS	N° nodes: NS DM:NS CRM:NS
Trastulli et al. (2011) [48]	8	854	-	NS	Favors R	Favors R	NS	N°nodes: NS DM:NS CRM:NS

R, robotic; L, laparoscopic; *NS*, non-significant; *DM*, distal margin; *CRM*, circumferential margin.

tion of the surgical specimen after very low or intersphincteric resection, due to doubts (now clarified) as to a possible increase of the risk of local relapse.

On the other hand, new techniques based on the use of either TEM or SILS instruments have emerged, both to tackle the technical difficulty of a very low rectal section in patients with bulky tumors in a narrow pelvis, and to facilitate distal rectum mobilization. This technical evolution might make it possible in future to overcome the "gray zone" 3 to 5 cm from the anal verge and perform the section safely from an oncological standpoint, both in laparoscopic and open surgery [54], even though its current application still awaits definition.

13.3 Surgical Strategies

For high rectal or intraperitoneal tumors, the surgical strategy is the same as has already been described, with very few exceptions, because postoperative complications and medium-long term consequences are few. Independently of whether neoadjuvant treatment is indicated or not, anterior resection (AR) remains the recommended choice in literature, whatever access is preferred.

In extraperitoneal low rectal tumors, the issues of oncological radicality and complications need to be considered. These have been already examined in previous chapters, and we mention them again here only in connection with strategic choices. If, until a few years ago, the discussion was based only on the best technical method for lowering the resection and reducing the distal clearance, today the therapeutic strategy includes the accuracy of imaging studies and the response to neoadjuvant therapy. The more debatable aspects are examined below.

13.3.1 Early Rectal Cancer

Early patterns of rectal cancer have been frequent in recent years, mostly in countries with a colorectal cancer screening program. The metastatic risk of initial tumors is well coded and for early tumors, confined within the submucosal layer, is close to 0; confirmation by transrectal ultrasound must be provided before these tumors can be treated, by local exeresis only, now carried out mainly with the TEM technique [55]. As already mentioned, a study aimed at identifying and assessing the role of the sentinel lymph node, possibly by laparoscopic sampling [56], is still ongoing: if this method is validated, with certainty of its negative predictive value, transanal techniques can also be used for T1 tumors greater than 4 cm or poorly differentiated, in which the lymph node metastatic risk is about 10% [57].

13.4 Integrated Role of the Neoadjuvant Therapy

13.4.1 Surgery after Complete Pathological Response

The current standard of neoadjuvant radio-chemotherapy (RCT) has introduced a new prognostic factor: histopathological regression after therapy, also called pathological complete response (pCR). This term refers to a response from both the primitive tumor and lymph node metastasis, which occurs in 10-15% of cases, as in our experience; however, it should be said that the pCR is not clearly defined in literature and varies from a simple volumetric assessment with magnetic resonance imaging (MRI) [58], to the use of multiparameter scores which include clinical and laboratory findings, and metabolic information, including CEA level and PET scan [59]. The Habr-Gama study shows a survival rate of patients with pCR, even without operation, similar to that of patients who had surgery, although the study was not randomized [60]. This data prompted a major discussion, not only as regards early tumors but also more advanced ones, even when there has been regression after RCT, as this strategy cancels the risks and complications of open or laparoscopic low rectal surgery [61]. A recent meta-analysis confirmed in an important number of patients that pCR is obtained in 15% of patients and is associated with a better oncological outcome [62]. At present most European authors recommend the execution of a full thickness biopsy or a transanal exeresis of the tumor zone after pCR in low rectal tumors [63, 64], only to confirm the clinical or radiological data; incidentally, no imaging method currently permits an absolute demonstration of the pCR. In the case of an incomplete response early conventional surgical treatment is recommended, without any worsening of the oncological outcome [65]. To confirm this approach, which no longer involves "sphincter saving surgery" but rather "rectal saving surgery", the CARTS [66] trial is ongoing. It aims to recruit patients with pCR (approximately 10-20% of cases) and offer them a TEM; if this procedure confirms the pCR histologically, the patients are merely referred to follow-up care, whereas if the tumor persists, they are sent for a surgical resection. The results of this kind of study will allow the validation of an even more conservative approach torectal cancer, no longer based only on imaging but also on the response to the therapy.

13.4.2 Tumors Requiring Resection at the First Diagnosis

As already reported in the chapter on resections, recommendations for abdominoperineal resection (APR) have gradually decreased over the years: initially indicated for tumors of the extraperitoneal rectum in the 1960s, the operation was then recommended for those under 6 cm from the anal verge in the 80s, for suprasphincteric ones in the 1990s, and finally for those with partial infiltration of the internal anal sphincter in the last decade. At the same time, and paradoxically, resection technique has undergone a number of modifications, such as greater lateral extension, because the classical operation left a significant risk of local relapse [67, 68], especially with a very low localization of the cancer. Consequently, it is difficult to decide precisely which patients to indicate for an APR, since the contraindications to a sphincter-saving resection (SSR) depend on the site of the tumor, the patient's morphology, his continence, and the surgeon's experience , as well as the difficulty of radiologic staging at this level.

The great majority of authors tend to reconsider the surgical indications after RCT, which means that some patients initially earmarked for APR can be treated with SSR after downsizing [69, 70], as long as the resection is R0 [71]. In this context, in case of doubts regarding CRM tumor involvement, or in case of difficulties in distinguishing between tumoral residue and post RT fibrosis, the patient may be a candidate for IORT, although this technology is not widespread [72]. Multicentric studies [73-75] do not clearly confirm this hypothesis, although it is difficult to extrapolate which patients are initially eligible for APR. However, Sauer [73] demonstrated that in patients initially elected for APR, 39% undergoing preoperative RCT could benefit from SSR, while this rate fell to 19% in those treated with postoperative RCT. Gérard [76] showed that a more complete pCR could be obtained by using preoperative RCT versus RT alone (11.4% vs. 3.6%), with a reduction in local recurrence rate (8.1% vs. 16.5%); despite these results, he did not demonstrate an improvement either in sphincter-saving procedures or in overall survival. Furthermore, it is not yet clear what is the best timing between RCT and surgery, although there is a tendency to extend the range from 4-6 to at least 8-10 weeks [75, 77].

The GRECCAR I trial demonstrated that 85% of patients initially eligible for APR could have been treated with SSR after restaging, three times out of four however with intersphincteric resection [78], which has debatable functional results. We agree with Rouanet that it does not seem ethically possible to propose a randomized clinical trial to compare APR versus SSR for tumors regressing after RCT [69].

Nevertheless it would seem reasonable to propose a plan of treatment tailored to these difficult cases, based on an assessment of the patient, age, morphology, continence, response to RCT, and also clinical, morphological and maybe biological and molecular parameters [79, 80] in view of the outcomes that can be achieved today with SSR; using anti-EGFR or antiangiogenics could be attractive, selecting the treatment according to K-ras mutation status [81].

An attempt to find a decision-making algorithm is set out in Figure 13.2.

How can we further improve oncological results in rectal cancers? Some authors advocate a better and more specific biological pretherapeutic characterization of the tumor, allowing the selection of more targeted drugs [82]. A hyper-fractionated, increased dose of radiotherapy was proposed in the Polish trial, with a possible increase in pCR [83]. On the other hand, no advantage seems to be gained by increasing or changing current patterns of chemotherapy

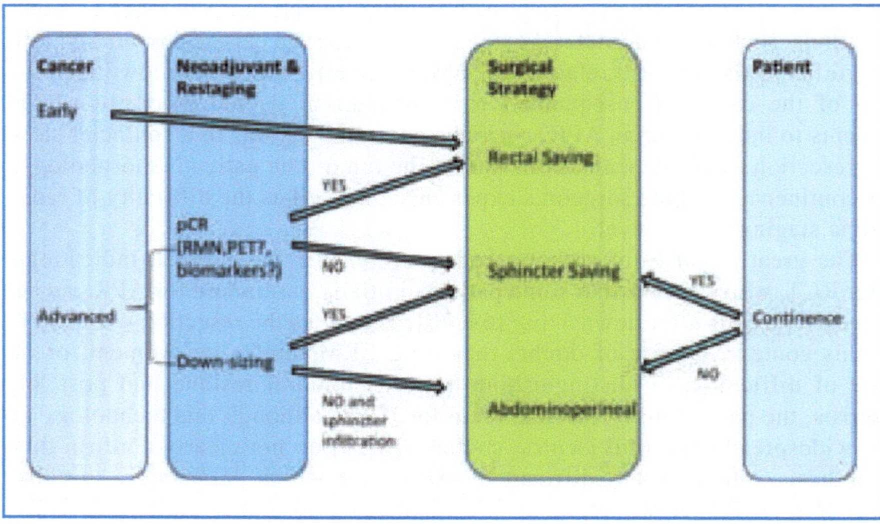

Fig. 13.2 Factors influencing surgical strategy in rectal cancer: patient characteristics, cancer stage, response to RCT

[84-88], though a better combination of drugs, radiotherapy, timing and interval between neoadjuvant treatment and surgery might be validated in the future. At present, in the absence of a specific individual prognostic marker, a statistical nomogram simply taking account of multiple factors could be used to establish a tailored treatment program [89].

In conclusion, the surgical strategy in rectal carcinoma has become particularly complex in the last few years, thanks to improvements in imaging, rapid evolution of surgical techniques, and new prognostic parameters such as pathological response. These tumor-linked factors combine with patient-related parameters like age, morphology and continence. While there is a general tendency to reduce surgical trauma and use a multimodal approach, there is not yet a worldwide consensus on many aspects of the therapeutic strategy for rectal carcinoma [90, 91], which tends to be connected to individual experience and the technology available in each center. Creation of a multidisciplinary plan is thus vital, perhaps concentrating treatment for this disease in high volume centers or, at least, in centers equipped to offer a multidisciplinary approach to rectal cancer.

References

1. Jayne DG, Guillou PJ, Thorpe H et al (2007) Randomized trial of laparoscopic-assisted resection of colorectal carcinoma: 3-year results of the UK MRC CLASICC Trial Group. J Clin Oncol 25:3061-3061

2. Fleshman J, Sargent DJ, Green E for The Clinical Outcomes of Surgical Therapy Study Group (2007) Laparoscopic colectomy for cancer is not inferior to open surgery based on 5-year data from the COST Study Group trial. Ann Surg 246:655-662
3. Veldkamp R, Kuhry E, Hop WC et al; COlon cancer Laparoscopic or Open Resection Study Group (COLOR) (2005) Laparoscopic surgery versus open surgery for colon cancer: short-term outcomes of a randomised trial. Lancet Oncol 6:477-484
4. Laurent C, Rullier E (2009) Place de la laparoscopie dans le traitement du cancer du rectum. In: Faucheron JL, Rullier E (eds) Cancer du rectum. Arnette, Wolter Kluwer France, pp 88-93
5. Morino M, Allaix ME, Giraudo G et al (2005) Laparoscopic versus open surgery for extraperitoneal rectal cancer: a prospective comparative study. Surg Endosc 19:1460-1467
6. Braga M, Frasson M, Vignali A et al (2007) Laparoscopic resection in rectal cancer patients: outcome and cost-benefit analysis. Dis Colon Rectum 50:464-471
7. Ströhlein MA, Grützner KU, Jauch KW, Heiss MM (2008) Comparison of laparoscopic vs. open access surgery in patients with rectal cancer: a prospective analysis. Dis Colon Rectum 51:385-391
8. Laurent C, Leblanc F, Wütrich P et al (2009) Laparoscopic versus open surgery for rectal cancer: long-term oncologic results. Ann Surg 250:54-61
9. Park J, Choi GS, Lim KH (2009) Laparoscopic resection of extraperitoneal rectal cancer: a comparative analysis with open resection. Surg Endosc 23:1818-1824
10. Kang SB, Park JW, Jeong SY et al (2010) Open versus laparoscopic surgery for mid or low rectal cancer after neoadjuvant chemoradiotherapy (COREAN trial): short-term outcomes of an open-label randomised controlled trial. Lancet Oncol 11:637-45
11. de Manzini N et al (2012) Unpublished data
12. Yamamoto S, Fukunaga M, Miyajima N et al; Japane Society of Laparoscopic Colorectal Surgery (2009) Impact of conversion on surgical outcomes after laparoscopic operation for rectal carcinoma: a retrospective study of 1,073 patients. J Am Coll Surg 208:383-389
13. Park IJ, Choi GS, Lim KH et al (2009)Multidimensional analysis of the learning curve for laparoscopic colorectal surgery: lessons from 1 000 cases of laparoscopic colorectal surgery. Surg Endosc 23:839-846
14. Rottoli M, Bona S, Rosati R et al (2009) Laparoscopic rectal resection for cancer: effects of conversion on short-term outcome and survival. Ann Surg Oncol 16:1279-1286
15. Targarona EM, Balague C, Pernas JC (2008) Can we predict immediate outcome after laparoscopic rectal surgery? Multivariate analysis of clinical, anatomic, and pathologic features after 3-dimensional reconstruction of the pelvic anatomy. Ann Surg 247:642-649
16. Veenhof AA, Engel AF, van der Peet DL et al (2008) Technical difficulty grade score for the laparoscopic approach of rectal cancer: a single institution pilot study. Int J Colorectal Dis 23:469-475
17. D'Hoore A, Wolthuis AM (2011) Laparoscopic low anterior resection and transanal pull-through for low rectal cancer: a Natural Orifice Specimen Extraction (NOSE) technique. Colorectal Dis 7:28-31
18. Zhou ZG, Hu M, Li Y (2004) Laparoscopic versus open total mesorectal excision with anal sphincter preservation for low rectal cancer.Surg Endosc 18:1211-1215
19. Påhlman L, Glimelius B, Frykholm G (1989) Ischaemic strictures in patients treated with a low anterior resection and perioperative radiotherapy for rectal carcinoma. Br J Surg 76:605-606
20. Aziz O, Constantinides V, Tekkis PP et al (2006) Laparoscopic versus open surgery for rectal cancer: a meta-analysis. Ann Surg Oncol 13:413-424
21. Varela JE, Wilson SE, Nguyen NT (2010) Laparoscopic surgery significantly reduces surgical-site infections compared with open surgery. Surg Endosc 24:270-276
22. Dobson MW, Geisler D, Fazio V et al (2011) Minimally invasive surgical wound infections: laparoscopic surgery decreases morbidity of surgical site infections and decreases the cost of wound care. Colorectal Dis 13:811-815

23. Laurent C, Leblanc F, Bretagnol F et al (2008)Long-term wound advantages of the laparoscopic approach in rectal cancer. Br J Surg 95:903-908
24. Panis Y, Maggiori L, Caranhac G et al (2011) Mortality after colorectal cancer surgery: a French survey of more than 84,000 patients. Ann Surg 254:738-743
25. Scarpa M, Erroi F, Ruffolo C (2009) Minimally invasive surgery for colorectal cancer: quality of life, body image, cosmesis, and functional results. Surg Endosc 23:577-582
26. Breukink S, Pierie J, Wiggers T (2006) Laparoscopic versus open total mesorectal excision for rectal cancer. Cochrane Database Syst Rev CD005200
27. Quah HM, Jayne DG, Eu KW, Seow-Choen F (2002) Bladder and sexual dysfunction following laparoscopically assisted and conventional open mesorectal resection for cancer. Br J Surg 89:1551-1556
28. Breukink SO, van Driel MF, Pierie JP (2008) Male sexual function and lower urinary tract symptoms after laparoscopic total mesorectal excision. Int J Colorectal Dis 23:1199-1205
29. Morino M, Parini U, Allaix ME et al (2009) Male sexual and urinary function after laparoscopic total mesorectal excision. Surg Endosc 23:1233-1240
30. Sartori CA, Sartori A, Vigna S et al (2011)Urinary and sexual disorders after laparoscopic TME for rectal cancer in males. J Gastrointest Surg 15:637-643
31. Trastulli S, Cirocchi R, Listorti C (2012) Laparoscopic versus open resection for rectal cancer: a meta-analysis of randomized clinical trials. Colorectal Dis [Epub ahead of print]
32. Rottoli M, Stocchi L, Geisler DP, Kiran RP (2012) Laparoscopic colorectal resection for cancer: effects of conversion on long-term oncologic outcomes. Surg Endosc [Epub ahead of print]
33. Kang SB, Park JS, Kim DW, Lee TG (2010). Intraoperative technical difficulty during laparoscopy-assisted surgery as a prognostic factor for colorectal cancer. Dis Colon Rectum 53:1400-1408
34. Reilly WT, Nelson H, Schroeder G (1996) Wound recurrence following conventional treatment of colorectal cancer. A rare but perhaps underestimated problem. Dis Colon Rectum 39:200-207
35. Jayne DG, Thorpe HC, Copeland J (2010) Five-year follow-up of the Medical Research Council CLASICC trial of laparoscopically assisted versus open surgery for colorectal cancer. Br J Surg 97:1638-1645
36. Bretagnol F, Dedieu A, Zappa M et al (2011) T4 colorectal cancer: is laparoscopic resection contraindicated? Colorectal Dis 13:138-143
37. van der Zaag ES, Buskens CJ, Vlug MS et al (2011) Decreased incidence of isolated tumor cells in lymph nodes after laparoscopic resection for colorectal cancer. Surg Endosc 25:3652-3657
38. Buunen M, Bonjer HJ, Hop WC, Haglind E et al (2009) COLOR II. A randomized clinical trial comparing laparoscopic and open surgery for rectal cancer. Dan Med Bull 56:89-91
39. Allaix ME, Degiuli M, Giraudo G et al (2012) Laparoscopic versus open colorectal resections in patients with symptomatic stage IV colorectal cancer. Surg Endosc [Epub ahead of print]
40. Bretagnol F, Hatwell C, Farges O et al (2008) Benefit of laparoscopy for rectal resection in patients operated simultaneously for synchronous liver metastases: preliminary experience. Surgery 144:436-441
41. Neugebauer EA, Becker M, Buess GF et al; European Association for Endoscopic Surgery (EAES) (2010) EAES recommendations on methodology of innovation management in endoscopic surgery. Surg Endosc 24:1594-615
42. Bianchi P, Petz W, Spinoglio G et al (2011) Robotic rectal resection in rectal cancer: short term results in an monocentric prospective study. Minerva Chir 66:527-535
43. Baek JH, Pastor C, Pigazzi A (2011) Robotic and laparoscopic total mesorectal excision for rectal cancer: a case-matched study. Surg Endosc 25:521-525
44. Kim NK, Kang J (2010) Optimal Total Mesorectal Excision for Rectal Cancer: the Role of Robotic Surgery from an Expert's View. J Korean Soc Coloproctol 26:377-387
45. Rawlings AL, Woodland JH, Vegunta RK, Crawford DL (2007) Robotic versus laparoscopic colectomy. Surg Endosc 21:1701-1708

46. Leong QM, Kim SH (2011) Robot-assisted rectal surgery for malignancy: a review of current literature.Ann Acad Med Singapore 40:460-466
47. Lin S, Jiang HG, Chen ZH et al (2011) Meta-analysis of robotic and laparoscopic surgery for treatment of rectal cancer.World J Gastroenterol 17:5214-5220
48. Trastulli S, Farinella E, Cirocchi R (2012) Robotic resection compared with laparoscopic rectal resection for cancer: systematic review and meta-analysis of short-term outcome. Colorectal Dis 14:e134-e156
49. Collinson FJ, Jayne DG, Pigazzi A (2012) An international, multicentre, prospective, randomised, controlled, unblinded, parallel-group trial of robotic-assisted versus standard laparoscopic surgery for the curative treatment of rectal cancer. Int J Colorectal Dis 27:233-241
50. Bulut O, Nielsen CB, Jespersen N (2011) Single-port access laparoscopic surgery for rectal cancer: initial experience with 10 cases. Dis Colon Rectum 54:803-809
51. Gaujoux S, Bretagnol F, Au J et al (2011) Single port access proctectomy with total mesorectal excision and intersphincteric resection with a primary transanal approach. Colorectal Dis 13:e305-307
52. Morino M, Verra M, Famiglietti F, Arezzo A (2011) Natural orifice transluminal endoscopic surgery (NOTES) and colorectal cancer? Colorectal Dis 7:47-50
53. Sylla P, Rattner DW, Delgado S, Lacy AM (2010) NOTES transanal rectal cancer resection using transanal endoscopic microsurgery and laparoscopic assistance. Surg Endosc 24:1205-1210
54. Wolthuis AM, Cini C, Penninckx F, D'Hoore A (2012) Transanal single port access to facilitate distal rectal mobilization in laparoscopic rectal sleeve resection with hand-sewn coloanal anastomosis. Tech Coloproctol 16:161-165
55. Tsai BM, Finne CO, Nordenstam JF et al (2010) Transanal endoscopic microsurgery resection of rectal tumors: outcomes and recommendations. Dis Colon Rectum 53:16-23
56. Cahill RA, Perretta S, Forgione A et al (2009) Multimedia article. Combined sentinel node biopsy and localized sigmoid resection entirely by natural orifice transluminal endoscopic surgery: a new challenge to the old paradigm. Dis Colon Rectum 52:725
57. Perretta S, Guerrero V, Garcia-Aguilar J (2006) Surgical treatment of rectal cancer: local resection. Surg Oncol Clin N Am 15:67-93
58. Nougaret S, Rouanet P, Molinari N et al (2012) MR Volumetric Measurement of Low Rectal Cancer Helps Predict Tumor Response and Outcome after Combined Chemotherapy and Radiation Therapy. Radiology 263:409-418
59. Park CH, Kim HC, Cho YB (2011) Predicting tumor response after preoperative chemoradiation using clinical parameters in rectal cancer. World J Gastroenterol 17:5310-5316
60. Habr-Gama A, Perez RO, Nadalin W (2004) Operative versus nonoperative treatment for stage 0 distal rectal cancer following chemoradiation therapy: long-term results. Ann Surg 240:711-717
61. Habr-Gama A, Perez R, Proscurshim I, Gama-Rodrigues J (2010) Complete clinical response after neoadjuvant chemoradiation for distal rectal cancer. Surg Oncol Clin N Am 19:829-845
62. Zorcolo L, Rosman AS, Restivo A et al (2012) Complete Pathologic Response after Combined Modality Treatment for Rectal Cancer and Long-Term Survival: A Meta-Analysis.Ann Surg Oncol [Epub ahead of print]
63. Rouanet P (2011) Complete response for rectal carcinoma after neoadjuvant therapy: to operate or not to operate? Surgeon's view Bull Cancer 98:25-29
64. Kennelly RP, Heeney A, White A (2011) A prospective analysis of patient outcome following treatment of T3 rectal cancer with neo-adjuvant chemoradiotherapy and transanal excision. Int J Colorectal Dis [Epub ahead of print]
65. Bujko K, Richter P, Kołodziejczyk M et al; Polish Colorectal Study Group [2009] Preoperative radiotherapy and local excision of rectal cancer with immediate radical re-operation for poor responders. Radiother Oncol 92:195-201
66. Bökkerink GM, de Graaf EJ, Punt CJ et al (2011) The CARTS study: Chemoradiation therapy for rectal cancer in the distal rectum followed by organ-sparing transanal endoscopic microsurgery. BMC Surg 11:34

67. West NP, Anderin C, Smith KJ, Holm T, Quirke P; European Extralevator Abdominoperineal Excision Study Group (2010) Multicentre experience with extralevator abdominoperineal excision for low rectal cancer. Br J Surg 97:588-599
68. Dalton RS, Smart NJ, Edwards TJ et al (2011) Short-term outcomes of the prone perineal approach for extra-levator abdomino-perineal excision (elAPE). Surgeon [Epub ahead of print]
69. Rouanet P (2009) Impact des traitements néo-adjuvants sur la conservation sphinctérienne des cancers du bas rectum. In Cancer du rectum. Faucheron JL, Rullier E (eds) Arnette, Paris, pp 80-87
70. Denost Q, Laurent C, Paumet T et al (2012) Laparoscopic surgery for rectal cancer: preoperative radiochemotherapy versus surgery alone. Surg Endosc [Epub ahead of print]
71. Marijnen CA, Nagtegaal ID, Kapiteijn E et al; Cooperative investigators of the Dutch Colerectal Cancer Group (2003) Radiotherapy does not compensate for positive resection margins in rectal cancer patients: report of a multicenter randomized trial. Int J Radiat Oncol Biol Phys 55:1311-1320
72. Dubois JB, Bussieres E, Richaud P et al (2011) Intra-operative radiotherapy of rectal cancer: results of the French multi-institutional randomized study.Radiother Oncol 98:298-303
73. Sauer R (2011) Preoperative versus postoperative chemoradiotherapy for locally advanced rectal cancer: results of the German CAO/ARO/AIO-94 randomized phase III trial after a median follow-up of 11 years. J Clin Oncol 29 (suppl) abs 3516
74. Roh MS, Colangelo LH, O'Connell MJ et al (2009) Preoperative multimodality therapy improves disease-free survival in patients with carcinoma of the rectum: NSABP R-03. J Clin Oncol 27:5124-5130
75. Pettersson D, Cedermark B, Holm T et al (2010) Interim analysis of the Stockholm III trial of preoperative radiotherapy regimens for rectal cancer. Br J Surg 97:580-587
76. Gérard JP, Conroy T, Bonnetain F et al (2006) Preoperative radiotherapy with or without concurrent fluorouracil and leucovorin in T3-4 rectal cancers: results of FFCD 9203. J Clin Oncol 24:4620-4625
77. Wolthuis AM, Penninckx F, Haustermans K et al (2012) Impact of Interval between Neoadjuvant Chemoradiotherapy and TME for Locally Advanced Rectal Cancer on Pathologic Response and Oncologic Outcome. Ann Surg Oncol [Epub ahead of print]
78. Rouanet P, Rivoire M, Lelong B et al (2006) Sphincter preserving surgery after preoperative treatment for ultralow rectal carcinoma. A French Multicenter prospective trial: GRECCAR I. ASCO Meeting Abstract 24 (Suppl) 3527
79. Deschoolmeester V, Boeckx C, Baay M (2010) KRAS mutation detection and prognostic potential in sporadic colorectal cancer using high-resolution melting analysis. Br J Cancer 103:1627-1636
80. Eberhard J, Gaber A, Wangefjord S et al (2012) A cohort study of the prognostic and treatment predictive value of SATB2 expression in colorectal cancer. Br J Cancer 106:931-938
81. Gérard JP, Francois E, Deustch E (2009) Neoadjuvant approach for non-metastatic rectal cancer combining radiotherapy and chemotherapy. Biotargeted drugs. Bull Cancer 96:321-328
82. Kim DW, Lim SB, Kim DYet al (2006) Pre-operative chemo-radiotherapy improves the sphincter preservation rate in patients with rectal cancer located within 3 cm of the anal verge. Eur J Surg Oncol 32:162–167
83. Bujko K, Nowacki MP, Nasierowska-Guttmejer A (2006) Long-term results of a randomized trial comparing preoperative short-course radiotherapy with preoperative conventionally fractionated chemoradiation for rectal cancer. Br J Surg 93:1215-1223
84. Gerard JP, Rostom Y, Gal J, Benchimol D et al (2012) Can we increase the chance of sphincter saving surgery in rectal cancer with neoadjuvant treatments: lessons from a systematic review of recent randomized trials. Crit Rev Oncol Hematol 81:21-28
85. Aschele C, Cionini L, Lonardi S et al (2011) Primary tumor response to preoperative chemoradiation with or without oxaliplatin in locally advanced rectal cancer: pathologic results of the STAR-01 randomized phase III trial. J Clin Oncol 29:2773-2780
86. Velenik V, Ocvirk J, Music M et al (2011) Neoadjuvant capecitabine, radiotherapy, and bevacizumab (CRAB) in locally advanced rectal cancer: results of an open-label phase II study. Radiat Oncol 6:105

87. Lim YK, Law WL, Liu R et al (2010) Impact of neoadjuvant treatment on total mesorectal excision for ultra-low rectal cancers. World J Surg Oncol 8:23
88. Bonnetain F, Bosset JF, Gerard JP et al (2012) What is the clinical benefit of preoperative chemoradiotherapy with 5FU/leucovorin for T3-4 rectal cancer in a pooled analysis of EORTC 22921 and FFCD 9203 trials: Surrogacy in question? Eur J Cancer [Epub ahead of print]
89. Valentini V, van Stiphout RG, Lammering G (2011)Nomograms for predicting local recurrence, distant metastases, and overall survival for patients with locally advanced rectal cancer on the basis of European randomized clinical trials. J Clin Oncol 29:3163-3172
90. Augestad KM, Lindsetmo RO, Stulberg J et al; International Rectal Cancer Study Group (IRCSG) (2010) International preoperative rectal cancer management: staging, neoadjuvant treatment, and impact of multidisciplinary teams. World J Surg 34:2689-2700
91. Siegel R, Cuesta MA, Targarona E et al; European Association for Endoscopic Surgery (EAES) (2011) Laparoscopic extraperitoneal rectal cancer surgery: the clinical practice guidelines of the European Association for Endoscopic Surgery (EAES). Surg Endosc 25:2423-2440

Surveillance after Curative Resection of Rectal Cancer

14

Piera Leon, Silvia Palmisano, Simonetta Masaro
and Nicolò de Manzini

14.1 Introduction

In the natural history of colorectal cancer, recurrence involves 30 to 50% of patients who have undergone curative surgical treatment [1] and occurs, in over 90% of cases, in the first 5 years following exeresis of the primitive tumor [2].

The risk of tumor recurrence is greater in patients presenting at diagnosis with a higher tumor stage (according to the commonly used TNM staging proposed by the American Joint Committee on Cancer, AJCC).

The most common sites of colorectal recurrence are, in order, liver (30-40%), lungs and locoregional relapse, with a highly variable incidence among the series of cases available.

The onset of another primitive colorectal tumor is also possible, and involves 3% of patients in the surveillance program [3].

The metachronous onset of metastasis, defined as secondary tumor sites diagnosed twelve months after surgical resection of the primary colorectal tumor, is the most frequent form of recurrence of the disease [4].

The liver is the first parenchymatous site of drainage, and is the organ most affected, through the portal venous system, by the hematic spread of the tumor located in the colorectal area.

The closer they are to the anal canal, rectal cancers, in particular, spread either to liver or to lungs, or both [5].

Metachronous metastases can also be located in other parts of the body, such as bones, brain, and potentially any organ through the hematic and lymphatic diffusion of neoplastic cells.

P. Leon (✉)
Department of Medicine, Surgery and Health Sciences, General Surgery Unit,
Cattinara University Hospital,
Trieste, Italy
e-mail: lep_ita@hotmail.com

N. de Manzini (ed.), *Rectal Cancer*,
Updates in Surgery
DOI: 10.1007/978-88-470-2670-4_14, © Springer-Verlag Italia 2013

Local recurrence of rectal carcinoma is less common than systemic tumor diffusion, and in literature is reported to affect from 3 to 33% of patients undergoing curative treatment [6].

The risk of local recurrence of rectal tumors is greater than that of colonic ones, due to their distinctive manner of spreading to the nearby organs and pelvis through the linfo-hematic and nervous systems. In fact, in these rectal lesions the preservation of adjacent organs, vessels and nerve structures can compromise the radicality of the surgical treatment and can lead to an increased risk of local recurrence.

The introduction of TME (Total Mesorectal Excision) surgery has improved local control in the treatment of rectal carcinoma, and has resulted in a drastic reduction, lower than 12%, in the incidence of pelvic recurrence [7]. The association of neoadjuvant radio-chemotherapy to TME has led to a further improvement in local control, limiting the relapse rate of rectal cancer to 6% [8].

Rectal relapse usually occurs in the extra-parietal rectal site, especially in the presacral area. Less frequently, the recurrence grows on the anastomotic scar or anywhere in the intraparietal area [9].

Patients already treated for colorectal cancer also present an increased risk of being affected by a second neoplasia of the residual viscera. It is a risk that lasts for life and is estimated to increase by 0.35% per year [10].

Recurrence is generally clinically evident only at a late, advanced stage and is frequently not suitable for curative saving surgery, with consequently poor prognosis.

Curative treatment for recurrence is, however, possible at a very early stage, when the neoplasm still has a limited spread; this substantially improves the prognosis [6], with an increase in global and cancer-specific survival. Unfortunately, radical surgery for local relapse can be performed only in 30-48% of the cases followed in the surveillance program [11, 12].

As far as hepatic metastases are concerned, the treatment of choice is multimodal therapy including hepatic resection [4] and chemotherapy. By using these combined treatments a 5-year survival rate of 30-40% can be achieved [4, 13]. On the other hand, chemotherapy alone extends the average lifetime to less than two years in patients with hepatic secondary lesions, especially in association with monoclonal antibodies with molecular targeting (Cetuximab and Bevacizumab) [14]. No treatment at all leads to a poor prognosis, usually less than a year.

14.2 Rationale of the Follow-up

The main aim of surveillance after curative surgery for rectal cancer is the early detection of recurrence, so as to implement a therapeutic strategy that can improve prognosis.

There is scientific evidence that curative surgery for recurrence at an early stage may substantially improve survival [15].

We recommend that surgeons perform a surveillance program to make an optimum assessment of oncological and functional outcomes (anorectal, sexual and urinary sequels), as well as the onset of possible long-term complications such as anastomotic stenosis and incisional hernia, and evaluate the patient's quality of life [16].

Post-surgical tumor resection surveillance also has psychological importance, which should not be underestimated: a surveillance program may either be regarded as a positive support and reassure the patient, or it may have the negative effect of generating stress, anxiety and/or fear.

14.3 Recommendations and Follow-up Programs

Surveillance after curative rectal carcinoma resection is internationally recommended as an integral part of the correct treatment for this kind of neoplasia; and it focuses on stages AJCC I, II and III, corresponding to Dukes' stages A, B and C [9].

Postoperative surveillance is also recommended in patients treated for synchronous or metachronous hepatic metastases with radical curative-intent therapy: recurrence in these cases may occur up to 60-70% [17]. Disease-free survival in radical hepatic re-resection is about 25% at five years, similar to that of primary resection [17]. Surveillance should be extended for at least two years after removing the hepatic metastasis, which is the usual time frame when almost all secondary hepatic tumor recurrences occur.

The exclusion criteria in the follow-up program are the following: patients not treated with curative-intent therapy, those affected by in situ neoplasia (AJCC stage 0), and patients whose age or general clinical conditions would not permit a surgical operation in the event of neoplastic recurrence.

In literature, there is still no consensus about the exact surveillance program to implement after curative treatment of rectal cancer. Each authoritative international oncological society indicates a follow-up scheme [6, 18-22], characterized by significant differences (Table 14.1).

On the other hand, there is greater agreement about the most appropriate period of time for which the surveillance program is conducted: generally in the five years following exeresis of the primitive rectal neoplasia.

Furthermore, there is no consensus on the diagnostic exams that should be used in surveillance, what their correct timing should be, and the costs-benefits of the resources used [23].

The international guidelines on the follow-up of rectal carcinomas are based on scientific evidence and on expert opinion [24]. They recommend an intensive monitoring at least for the first three years after surgical resection, using clinical examinations, serum CEA (Carcino-Embryonic Antigen) level measures, radiological imaging investigations of abdomen and thorax, and endoscopic exams.

Table 14.1 International Guidelines on the follow-up of rectal carcinomas

Guideline	Clinic visit	Cea level	Abdominal imaging	Chest imaging	Colonoscopy
ASCO [18]	Every 3-6 mo for 3 y, then every 6 mo for 2 y, then at discretion of physician	Every 3 mo for 3 y or longer in patients stage II e III	CT annually for 3 y for patients stage II and III, extended to pelvis for rectal cancer (especially if not irradiated and with poor differentiation)	CT annually for 3 y	Perioperative, then at 3 y, then every 5 y. Proctosigmoidoscopy every 6 mo in rectal cancer stage II and III not irradiated
ASCRS [6]	Every 3 mo for 2 y	Every 3 mo for 2 y	Not recommended	Not recommended	At 1 y, then every 3-5 y, periodic proctosigmoidoscopy in rectal cancer stage II e III not irradiated
ESMO [19]	Every 3-6 mo for 3 y, then for 6-12 mo for 2 y	Every 3-6 mo for 3 y, then for 6-12 mo for 2 y	Liver US every 6 mo for 3 y, then annually for 2 y; CT annually for 3 y in high-risk patients	CRX annually for 5 y; CT annually for 3 y in high risk patients	At 1 y, then every 3-5 y, proctosigmoidoscopy every 6 mo for 2 y in nonirradiated rectal cancer
NCCN [20]	Every 3-6 mo for 2 y, then every 6 mo for 5 y	Every 3-6 mo for 2 y, then every 6 mo for 5 y for T2 or more	CT abdomen and pelvis annually for 3 y in high risk patients (poor differentiation)	Not recommended	At 1, 3 and 5 y; proctosigmoidoscopic evaluation every 6 mo for 5 y in post-LAR nonirradiated rectal cancer
NHS [21]	Not specified	Not recommended	CT o Liver US within 2 y	Not recommended	Within first y, then as indicated by the surgeon
CCO [22]	Every 6 mo for 3 y, then every y for 5 y	At surgeon's discretion	Liver US at surgeon's discretion	CRX at surgeon's discretion	Colonoscopy periodic long-life; proctosigmoidoscopic evaluation every 6 mo for 5 y

ASCO, American Society of Clinical Oncology; *ASCRS*, American Society of Colon and Rectal Surgeons; *ESMO*, European Society for Medical Oncology; *NCCN*, National Comprehensive Cancer Network (US); *NHS*, National Health Service (UK); *CCO*, Cancer Care Ontario (CAN).

It is thought, but has not yet been clearly scientifically proven, that an intensive follow-up could lead to early detection of disease recurrence, subsequently permitting radical resection with an increase in global survival [25].

According to six randomized clinical studies out of eight [26-33], a high-intensity follow-up program does not improve survival in patients treated for rectal cancer.

Recently, however, some authors [16, 22, 34] highlighted an advantage in overall survival and a higher rate of preclinical diagnosis of resectable recurrence, but no cancer-specific survival was documented in the high intensity regime of surveillance [23].

Further investigations are, therefore, necessary to assess the real benefit in terms of survival of post-curative surgery surveillance for rectal carcinoma and to define the recommended follow-up scheme to be used.

Three large randomized clinical studies (RCT) [16] (Table 14.2) were recently performed to define the effectiveness and the features of correct post-operative surveillance in patients treated for rectal carcinoma with curative intent. The results, global and cancer-specific survival, quality of life and cost-benefits are not yet available.

14.4 Follow-up Modalities

14.4.1 Anamnesis and Clinical Examination

Anamnesis and clinical examination remain recommended instruments to be used in all follow-up programs, but they do not influence global survival rate [16].

Indeed, symptoms in rectal recurrence are often aspecific and are manifest too late to perform a curative resection, so the patient's outcome is usually poor [9].

The medical visit still remains a valid instrument for maintaining contact with the patient. It allows discussions of the results of the tests performed during the follow-up and of the need for further examinations if necessary; it also provides psychological support and leads to awareness of the trend of the disease.

Furthermore, the clinical examination may highlight functional outcomes and systemic toxicities as a consequence of multimodal curative treatment of rectal cancer, so that in some cases specific treatments aimed at improving or clearing them up can be given [23].

14.4.2 Measuring the Hematic Level of Cea

CEA is a fetal glycol-protein, which is physiologically produced and secreted during fetal life. It can also be synthetized during adulthood due to both benign and malign causes.

Table 14.2 On-going Randomized Clinical Trials

On-going RCT	GILDA	FACS-NCT00560365	COLOFOL-NCT00225641
Study start date	May 1998	March 2004	March 2006
Estimated study completion date		December 2013	December 2015
Inclusion criteria	CRC Dukes B2-C (R0)	Aged 50 or more, both genders, CRC AJCC I, II and III (R0)	Aged 18 to 75 year-old, both genders, CRC AJCC stage II, III (R0)
Estimated enrollment	2920	4760	2500
Study plan	Rectal cancer: 2 groups intensive vs minimalist follow-up regime Colon cancer: 2 groups, intensive vs minimalist follow-up regime	4 groups with increasingly intensive follow-up: Arm I: symptomatic follow-up Arm II: Cea serum level assessment scheduled Arm III: CT scan or MRI scheduled Arm IV: both arm II and III	2 groups with high vs. low intensive follow-up regime: Arm I: CT scan, CXR and Cea serum level scheduled Arm II: CT scan, CXR and Cea serum level at 12 and 36 mo from surgery
Locations	Italy	United Kingdom	Denmark, Sweden, Poland, Holland, Uruguay, Ireland
Outcome measures	Overall survival, Cancer-specific mortality, Treatment of recurrence, Sensitivity of follow-up regimen, Follow-up compliance, Quality of life	Overall survival, Quality of life, Costs, Cost per year-life saved	Overall survival, Cancer-specific mortality, Disease-free survival
Up-date	Fossati c/o Mario Negri Institute Milan, Italy	www.facs.soton.ac.uk	www.colofol.com

GILDA, Gruppo Italiano di Lavoro sulla Diagnosi Anticipata; a multicentre randomized trial of intensive vs. minimalist strategy in the follow-up of patients with resected Dukes B-C colorectal carcinoma; *FACS*, Follow-up after Colorectal cancer; a randomized controlled trial to assess the cost-effectiveness of Intensive versus No Scheduled Follow-up in patients who have undergone resection for colorectal cancer with curative intent;
COLOFOL, a pragmatic study to assess the frequency of surveillance tests after curative resection in patients with stage II and III colorectal cancer – a Randomized Multicentre Trial.

It is used as a tumor marker and is more useful in surveillance after exeresis of the rectal neoplasia than in preoperatory diagnostic assessment.

CEA is often the first marker of recurrence of the disease, appearing in the blood about 4.5-8 months before any clinical manifestation of recurrence [6, 15].

It increases in about half of the cases of neoplastic recurrence [8, 35], becoming as high as 75% in some cases studies [6, 9]. The postoperative hematic level increases even in recurrence of rectal cancer not producing CEA before exeresis.

Assessment of serum CEA level is widely recommended in follow-up programs for rectal carcinoma, although there is no scientific evidence that its measurement at regular intervals can improve survival or increase the resectability of the recurrence [35].

The sensitivity and specificity of its hematic level for disease recurrence is related to the cut-off value considered: a cut-off value of 10 UI/l has a sensitivity and specificity respectively of 44% and 90%, while with a value of 6 UI/l, sensitivity increases to 80% and specificity drops to 42%. The number of false positives with a cut-off value of 6 UI/l is high, as much as 7-16% [9, 23].

CEA is falsely increased in smokers [35] and in patients undergoing chemotherapy with fluoropyrimidine [18].

A three-time increase in the CEA value and an exceedance of the cut-off are both suggestive of disease recurrence.

CEA is more sensitive for hepatic and retroperitoneal recurrence, than for peritoneal and lung tumor spread [6, 9, 23].

Other laboratory tests, such as blood tests, and hepatic and renal function tests, are not routinely recommended [9].

14.4.3 Hepatic Imaging

Study of the hepatic parenchyma in the surveillance program for rectal cancer is justified by the high recurrence rate in this organ.

It has been demonstrated that laboratory hepatic function tests are not useful in the preclinical diagnosis of recurrence and are not, therefore, routinely recommended [6].

The international guidelines on follow-up programs advise radiological methods for studying the hepatic parenchyma: abdominal CT is generally preferred, hepatic ultrasound exam is chosen less often [19].

As published in literature, CT scan permits preclinical diagnoses of recurrence, but there is no agreement on the real advantages in terms of resection rate [9, 16, 23].

Abdominal CT scan has good sensitivity (64% according to Bipat [36], 78 to 100% according to other investigations [37]) in detecting secondary hepatic disease, but loses diagnostic accuracy in determining extra-hepatic disease (it shows high false negative rates in detecting the periaortic lymph nodes involved) [38].

Recent studies are concentrating on improving the diagnosis of liver metastases using hepatic perfusion and hepatic parenchyma texture measurements during CT scan examinations [39].

Liver ultrasound (US) has a lower sensitivity in diagnosing metastases than CT scanning [40]. Hepatic ultrasound, while sparing the patient from the effect of ionising radiation, is operator dependent and is not reliable regarding the detection of extra hepatic intra-abdominal recurrence.

The ASCRS (American Society of Colon and Rectal Surgeons) [6] does not routinely recommend the use of hepatic imaging, claiming that it rarely detects hepatic metastasis before CEA increase. In their opinion, the detection of liver metastases before CEA increase does not improve surgical resection rate. The use of liver imaging is recommended when suspicion of a secondary lesion is raised by an abnormal CEA test or clinical findings.

In literature, the survival advantage of the use of hepatic radiological imaging, even in intensive follow-up programs, is still controversial, and doubts remain as to whether it may be sustainable in terms of costs.

14.4.4 Lung Imaging

Recurrence after treatment of rectal carcinoma can also occur in the lungs. The frequency of metastases in the lungs increases the closer to the anal-verge the rectal carcinomas are, because of caval venous drainage of the very distal viscera.

Not all international guidelines recommend monitoring the lung parenchyma, but when the oncological societies suggest it, the lung parenchyma may be assessed by conventional X rays or by a CT scan.

Chest X ray (CRX) does not permit early diagnosis of disease relapse [6], does not affect the resection rate and does not modify survival.

Thorax CT scan has more diagnostic accuracy than traditional chest X rays and is the preferred investigation technique in the study of lung parenchyma [40]. It also still yields a fair number of false positives [38], as well as involving costs that are not negligible.

14.4.5 Endoscopic Examinations

The rationale of using endoscopic exams in follow-up programs is to detect anastomotic or intraparietal relapse and metachronous colorectal cancer.

Rectal cancers have a higher rate of local recurrence than colonic tumors. They actually frequently develop extra-parietally, usually in the posterior presacral site.

Patients with colorectal neoplasia treated surgically with curative intent present a cumulative risk of 3% every six years of being affected by a metachronous tumor in the residual viscera [23].

The risk of developing benign and malign metachronous tumors lasts for life, so the recommendation to perform a colonoscopy at regular intervals is not limited to the first years following exeresis.

Colonoscopy is a surveillance tool that all the major oncological societies recommend performing in the first, third and fifth year after surgery; its use has a wide consensus in literature [23].

Colonoscopy does not seem to improve the five-year survival rate [6, 40], probably due a lower rate of local recurrence than systemic spread, and to the more frequent extra-parietal presacral relapses among local recurrences.

The number of resectable recurrences diagnosed at colonoscopy varies considerably in literature, between 0 and 19% [40].

Many authoritative oncological societies [6, 18-20, 22] also recommend performing a proctosygmoidoscopy every 6 months for a period ranging from two and five years after the exeresis of the primitive rectal tumor in patients with a high risk of local relapse (AJCC stages II and III, patients who have not undergone neoadjuvant radiochemotherapy, and patients affected by cancer with poor prognostic histologic features).

Despite being a major test in the surveillance program, compliance to endoscopy is low compared to other techniques, often lower than 50% [40].

Some ongoing clinical studies are assessing the effectiveness of the use of rectal ecoendoscopy [9] for early diagnosis of local extra-parietal relapse in rectal cancer, although no results of clear cost-benefits have emerged so far.

Virtual colonoscopy, a topographic abdominal CT scan with multiplanar reconstructions of the colonic viscera, may be a promising alternative, overcoming the problem of invasiveness and patient compliance. Virtual colonoscopy seems to be able to determine both the presence of metachronous tumors and abdominal metastases [39]. However, it shows a considerable number of false positives, and does not allow histological sampling, which is useful in making a definitive carcinoma diagnosis

Fecal occult blood testing is not included in colorectal cancer surveillance because of the unquestionable need for colonoscopy [6].

14.4.6 Second-level Examinations

The main second-level exam in the study of rectal cancer recurrence is Positron Emission Tomography associated to a CT scan (PET/CT).

PET/CT highlights the tissue sites with higher glucose metabolism to determine the main areas of cell activity. Cell metabolism is typically high in neoplastic tissues but also in inflammatory sites, producing a limited amount of false positive cases.

PET/CT is recommended in the event of an increase in tumor markers and no evidence of recurrence both in radiological imaging and endoscopic exams.

It has a higher sensitivity than CT scan and Magnetic Resonance (MR) exams in diagnosing hepatic metastases (94%) as well as in diagnosing extrahepatic intra-abdominal and even extra-abdominal recurrence (sensitivity of 90-100%, greater than any other method) [40].

It permits a global assessment of the tumor spread, which is useful in planning the correct treatment strategy.

However, PET/CT is expensive and is not widespread, features that limit its routine use in the follow-up of rectal cancer.

The use of the super paramagnetic contrast agents SPIO (Super-Paramagnetic Iron Oxide) in Magnetic Resonance Imaging increases the sensitivity of MRI (76%) alone and looks promising for defining intra-abdominal neoplastic recurrence; however, it does not assess lung parenchyma, it is expensive, and currently it has limited availability [39].

14.5 Proposals for Molecular Studies

On-going clinical studies are assessing the effectiveness of new diagnostic exams in the context of surveillance programs.

The focus is on defining predictive factors of disease relapse, to determine which patients are at higher risk of recurrence.

Beside the well-known prognostic factors (stage, histological degree, number of lymph nodes analysed, vascular, neural and lymphatic invasion) [18], some molecular markers of neoplastic cells such as 18qLOH, c-myc, bcl-2, cell-suicide related genes, TGF, EGF, VEGF, receptors for somatostatin, L-catenin, MUC-1 mucin, proliferative indices like Ki-67, and DNA content are under investigation as to their ability to predict the individual risk of recurrence.

It is known that tumors presenting a marked instability of the microsatellites and wide methylation of anti-tumor genes tend to relapse as metachronous tumors in the residual viscera or as local recurrence rather than distant metastases: in these cases endoscopic surveillance increases in importance compared to other follow-up exams [40].

Stratifying the patients into risk levels means that tailored surveillance programs can be implemented, keeping costs down [40] and offering rates of high-intensity surveillance to patients at higher risk of recurrence and low-intensity surveillance to patients at lower risk of recurrence.

14.6 Conclusions

Postsurgical treatment surveillance is internationally recommended as part of the correct treatment for rectal cancer.

The main aim of surveillance after curative surgery is the early detection of possible relapses, so that therapeutic strategies that could improve prognosis can be implemented.

In fact, carcinoma recurrence is related to a poor prognosis affecting from a third to half of the patients treated initially with curative intent for localized and resectable rectal neoplasia. Relapse occurs in most cases within the first three years following the exeresis of the primitive lesion and in almost all cases within the first five years after primary tumor resection.

Surveillance is recommended for patients presenting at diagnosis in AJCC stages I, II and III, corresponding to Dukes' stages A, B and C.

Postoperative surveillance is also recommended in patients treated with curative intent for synchronous or metachronous hepatic metastases.

Patients excluded from follow-up are those not treated with curative intent, those affected by in situ neoplasia, and patients whose age or general clinical conditions would not permit surgical intervention in the event of tumor recurrence.

In literature, there is still no consensus on a single surveillance program, and debate is open about which diagnostic exams to use, frequency of their employment, cost-benefit, and real survival advantage. Discordant data regarding survival advantage have recently been published.

Three on-going multicentre trials (GILDA, FACS and COLOFOL) have been launched to define the correct surveillance program, the cost-benefit of a possible stratification of the patients according to the risk of recurrence, survival advantage deriving from an intensive follow-up regime. Results of these multicentre trials are not yet available.

References

1. Bohm B, Schwenk W, Hucke HP et al (1993) Does methodic long-term follow-up affect survival after curative resection of colorectal carcinoma? Dis Colon Rectum 36:280-286
2. Obrand D, Gordon P (1997) Incidence and patterns of recurrence following curative resection of colon cancer. Dis Colon Rectum 40:15-24
3. Galandiuk S, Wieand HS, Moertel CG et al (1992) Patterns of recurrence after curative resection of carcinoma of the colon and rectum. Surg Gynecol Obstet 174:27-32
4. Capussotti L (2011) Surgical treatment of colorectal liver metastases. Springer Verlag Edition
5. Tepper JE, O'Connell M, Niedzwiecki D et al (2002) Adjuvant therapy in rectal cancer: Analysis of stage, sex, and local control. Final report of Intergroup 0114. J Clin Oncol 20:1744-1750
6. Giordano P, Efron J, Vernava AM et al (2006) Strategies of follow-up for colorectal cancer: a survery of American Society of Colon and Rectal Surgeons. Tech Coloproctol 10:199-207
7. MacFarlane JK, Ryall RDH, Heald RJ (1993) Mesorectal excision for rectal cancer. Lancet 341:457-460
8. Kapiteijn E, Marijnen CAM, Nagtegaal ID et al (2001) Preoperative radiotherapy combined with total mesorectal excision for resectable rectal cancer. New Engl J Med 345:638-646
9. Anthony T, Simmang C, Hyman N et al (2004) Practice Parameters for the Surveillance and Follow-Up of Patients With Colon and Rectal Cancer. Dis Colon Rectum 47:807-817
10. Cali RL, Pitsch RM, Thorson A et al (1993) Cumulative incidence of metachronous colorectal cancer. Dis Colon Rectum 36:388-393
11. Lopez-Kostner F, Fazio VW, Vignali A et al (2001) Locally recurrent rectal cancer: predictors of success of salvage surgey. Dis Colon Rectum 44:173-178
12. Garcia Aguilar J, Cromwell JW, Marra C et al (2001) Treatment of locally recurrent rectal cancer. Dis Colon Rectum 41:1743-1748

13. Elias D, Sideris L, Pocard M et al (2004) Results of R0 resection for colorectal liver metastases associated with extrahepatic disease. Ann Surg Oncol 11:274-280
14. Kelly H, Goldberg RM (2005) Systemic therapy for metastatic colorectal cancer: current opinions, current evidence. J Clin Oncol 23:4553-60
15. Baca B, Beart RW, Etzioni DA (2011) Surveillance after colorectal cancer resection: a systematic review. Dis Colon Rectum 54:1036-1048
16. Jeffery M, Hickey BE, Hider PN (2007) Follow-up strategies for patients treated for non-metastatic colorectal cancer. Cochrane Database of Systematic Reviews 1 CD002200
17. Langenhoff BS, Krabbe PF, Ruers TJ (2009) Efficacy of follow-up after surgical treatment of colorectal liver metastases. Eur J Surg Oncol 35:180-186
18. Desch CE, Benson AB, Somerfield MR et al (2005) Colorectal cancer surveillance: 2005 update of an American Society of Clinical Oncology practice guidelines. J Clin Oncol 23:8512-8519
19. Van Cutsem EJ, Oliveira J (2008) Colon cancer: ESMO clinical recommendations for diagnosis, adjuvant treatment and follow-up. Ann Oncol 19:29-30
20. NCCN National Comprehensive Cancer Network (2009) Clinical Practice Guidelines in Oncology
21. Scholefield JH, Steele RJ (2002) Guidelines for follow-up after resection of colorectal cancer. Gut 51:V3-V5
22. Figueredo A, Rumble RB, Maroun J et al (2003) Follow-up of patients with curatively resected colorectal cancer: a practice guideline. BMC Cancer 3:26
23. Scheer A, Auer R (2009) Surveillance after curative resection of colorectal cancer. Clin Colon Rectal Surg 22:242-250
24. Fernandez SP, Diaz SP, Lopez Calvino B et al (2010) Diagnosis delay and follow-up strategies in colorectal cancer. Prognosis implications: a study protocol. BMC Cancer 10:528
25. Renehan AG, Egger M, Saunders MP et al (2002) Impact on survival of intensive follow-up after curative resection for colorectal cancer: systematic review and meta-analysis of randomized trials. BMJ 324:813
26. Makela JT, Laitinen SO, Kairaluoma MI (1995) Five-year follow-up after radical surgery for colorectal cancer. Results of a prospective randomized trial. Arch Surg 130:1062-1067
27. Ohlsson B, Breland U, Ekberg H et al (1995) Follow-up after curative surgery for colorectal carcinoma. Randomized comparison with no follow-up. Dis Colon Rectum 38:619-626
28. Kjeldsen BJ, Kronborg O, Fenger C et al (1997) A prospective randomized study of follow-up after radical surgery for colorectal cancer. Br J Surg 84:666-669
29. Pietra N, Sarli L, Costi R et al (1998) Role of follow-up in management of local recurrences of colorectal cancer: a prospective, randomized study. Dis Colon Rectum 41:1127-1133
30. Shoemaker D, Black R, Giles L et al (1998) Yearly colonoscopy, liver CT, and chest radiography do not influence 5-year survival of colorectal cancer patients. Gastroenterology 114:7-14
31. Secco GB, Fardelli R, Gianquinto D et al (2002) Efficacy and cost of risk-adapted follow-up in patients after colorectal cancer surgery: a prospective, randomized and controlled trial. Eur J Surg Oncol 28:418-423
32. Rodriguez-Moranta F, Salò J, Arcusa A et al (2006) Postoperative surveillance in patients with colorectal cancer who have undergone curative resection: a prospective, multicenter, randomized, controlled trial. J Clin Oncol 24:386-393
33. Grossmann EM, Johnson FE, Virgo KS et al (2004) Follow-up of colorectal cancer patients after resection with curative intent, the GILDA trial. Surg Oncol 13:119-124
34. Tjandra JJ, Chan MK (2007) Follow-up after curative resection of colorectal cancer: a meta-analysis. Dis Colon Rectum 50:1783-1799
35. Korner H, Soreide K, Stokkeland PJ et al (2006) Diagnostic accuracy of serum-carcinoembryonic antigen in Recurrent Colorectal Cancer: a receiver operating characteristic curve analysis. Annals of Surgical Oncology 4:417-423
36. Bipat S, van Leeuwen MS, Ijzermans JN et al (2007) Evidence based guidelines on management of colorectal liver metastases in the Netherlands. Net J Med 65:5-14

37. Patel S, McCall M, Ohinmaa A et al (2011) Position Emission Tomography/Computer Tomographic Scans compared to Computer Tomographic Scans for detecting colorectal liver metastases; a systematic review. Ann Surg 253:666-671
38. Maas M, Rutten IJG, Nelemans PJ et al (2011) What is the most accurate whole body imaging modality for assessment of local and distant recurrent disease in colorectal cancer? A meta-analysis. Eur J Nucl Med Mol Imaging 38:1560-1571
39. Miles K, Burkill G (2007) Colorectal cancer: imaging surveillance following resection of primary tumor. Cancer Imaging 7:S143-S149
40. Soreide K (2010) Endoscopic surveillance after curative surgery for sporadic colorectal cancer: patient-tailored, tumor-targeted or biology-driven? Scand J Gastroenterol 45:1255-1261

Treatment of Local Recurrence

15

Paola Graziotin and Nicolò de Manzini

15.1 Introduction

The incidence of local recurrence of rectal cancer after curative resection ranges from 2.6 to 32% [1] and is related to the stage of the primitive tumor and to the quality of the initial surgical treatment. Before the introduction of total mesorectal excision and neoadjuvant radiochemotherapy, around 80% of recurrences appeared within the first 2 years of surgery with an average time of onset ranging between 6 and 12 months [2].

Neoadjuvant radiochemotherapy has contributed to the reduction of recurrence and extended disease-free survival. The current average relapse time ranges from 20 to 39 months after surgery and in about 24% of cases it occurs 5 years after the first operation [3].

The prognosis for patients with recurrence of rectal cancer is unfavorable. Five-year survival rate in the absence of treatment is less than 5%, with an average survival rate of 7 months [4]. 50% of patients with local recurrence do not have metastatic disease. The most frequent symptoms correlated to recurrence are pain due to nerve involvement, tenesmus, rectal bleeding and stenosis in endoluminal recurrence [5]. In patients not eligible for iterative surgery, these symptoms can be partially controlled by radio- and chemotherapy , which can extend survival up to 10-17 months.

The only treatment option remains surgical resection, associated or not to radio- and chemotherapy, even though it is not always technically feasible and is often associated with high morbidity and major changes in the patient's

P. Graziotin (✉)
Department of Medicine, Surgery and Health Sciences, General Surgery Unit,
Cattinara University Hospital,
Trieste, Italy
e-mail: polz1979@libero.it

N. de Manzini (ed.), *Rectal Cancer,*
Updates in Surgery
DOI: 10.1007/978-88-470-2670-4_15

quality of life. The curative resection rate (R0) in the various cases ranges from 30 to 45% [6], while the survival rates 5 years after iterative surgery range from 0 to 50% [7].

15.2 Diagnosis

Physical examination and, mostly, digital rectal exploration play an important role in the diagnosis of local recurrence, allowing intra- or extraluminal lesions to be identified and providing information about the degree of mobility or fixity of the lesion in the deep layers [8].

Intraluminal recurrence can be identified by rectosigmoidoscopy, while pancolonoscopy remains an important tool for excluding the presence of synchronous colonic tumors.

However, in most cases rectal cancer recurrence is extraluminal [9]. Transanal ultrasound makes it possible to identify the extraluminal recurrence, permitting execution of a guided biopsy, but provides limited information on the extent and resectability of the mass.

CT and MRI are comparable in terms of diagnostic accuracy and provide detailed information on the limits and extent of the neoplasia. Their only limitation is the difficulty of distinguishing recurrence from scar tissue in a pelvis treated with radiotherapy. PET is capable of confirming the presence of recurrence with a degree of diagnostic accuracy higher than CT and MRI and equal to 87%, whereas PET-CT has a sensitivity up to 100% and a specificity of 96% [10].

15.3 Classification of Recurrence

The classification of recurrence proposed by the Mayo Clinic is based on the patient´s symptoms (S0=asymptomatic, S1=symptomatic without pain, S2=symptomatic with pain), on the site where the mass is located on the pelvis (anterior, posterior, lateral right and lateral left), and on the number of sites of fixation to the pelvic wall (F0=0 points, F1=1 point, F2=2 points, F3= 3 points) [11].

Wanebo et al. proposed a classification based on the UICC TNM system. TR1 and TR2 are intraluminal recurrences on the primary resection site. TR3 is a recurrence at a deep anastomotic level, which reaches the perivisceral adipose tissue; TR4 describes the invasion of the adjacent organs (uterus, vagina, bladder, prostate, seminal vesicles) without penetration in the bone tissues; finally, TR5 describes the invasion of bony and ligamentous structures of the sacrum and of the lateral pelvic walls [12].

Yamada et al. classify recurrence on the basis of the fixing pattern on the pelvis into localized (adjacent to pelvic organs and connective tissue), sacral (S3-S5 level, coccygeal, limited to the periosteum) and lateral (lateral walls of the pelvis, sacrum at S1-S2 level, greater sciatic foramen, sciatic nerve). The infiltration pattern is a prognostic index with different 5-year survival rates, ranging from 38% in the localized forms, to 10% in the sacral and close to 0% in the lateral ones [13].

The classification of the Memorial Sloan-Kettering Cancer Center group includes axial, anterior, posterior and lateral recurrence. *Axial* recurrence can be divided into anastomotic, extending to the perivisceral tissue and perineal in patients undergoing abdominoperineal amputation; *anterior* recurrence involves the genitourinary tract, including uterus, vagina, bladder, prostate and seminal vesicles; *posterior* relapse means an involvement of the sacrum and presacral fascia, and *lateral* relapse affects the lateral soft tissue and vascular structures of the pelvis and the pelvic bones [14].

15.4 Selection Criteria for Surgery

The presence of distant metastases constitutes a contraindication to surgical treatment of the recurrence, since it would require invalidating operations with no curative purpose.

In highly selected cases, combined surgical treatment of the recurrence and metastases is possible [9].

If the recurrence is not treatable by radical surgery, palliative treatment can be given, as it can lower the patient's morbidity. Some authors claim that non-radical surgery can be justified in this setting, since the partial removal of the neoplastic mass can provide limited relief of the symptoms. However, this position is debatable, because R2 re-resections are often invalidating and give very short-term pain relief [15].

If there is a recurrence obstructing the rectal lumen, a stent should be placed; when stenting is not possible, then colostomy is indicated [16].

Radiotherapy is frequently the first choice for palliation, often in association with chemotherapy.

It has been demonstrated that RT can help to reduce symptoms like pain and bleeding and improve the quality of life of these patients [17].

Bleeding recurrences can be controlled by laser ablations or selective embolization.

Surgical treatment of resectable recurrences includes a heterogeneous group of procedures, which depend on the site and extent of the mass. The goal is to achieve an en-bloc removal of the mass with negative margins (R0). In fact, R0 resection is the only curative treatment, while R1 and R2 are merely palliative. It is thus clearly mandatory to select only patients who can benefit from an R0 intervention before performing demolition re-operations.

Major contraindications to re-resections are: extended circumferential or lateral involvement of the pelvis; infiltration of the iliac vessels with edema of the lower limbs; bilateral ureter infiltration with hydronephrosis; sciatic nerve infiltration with sciatica; metastasis to the para-aortic lymph nodes, and finally a limited infiltration of the sacrum and the lateral walls below S2 [9].

Surgical treatment may require a multidisciplinary team made up of a surgeon, urologist, orthopedist and radiotherapist. Placing ureteral stents in the preoperative setting can often help the operation.

Repeat surgery is not possible in 25 to 50% of cases, due to intraoperative findings of misrecognized metastases or advanced extent of the disease.

15.5 Adjuvant Therapy

Neoadjuvant treatment increases the number of cases in which a surgical resection with curative intent can be performed; moreover, it improves the outcomes, extending the 5-year overall survival and disease-free survival rates.

Patients who have not received preoperative radiotherapy can be subjected to a medium irradiation dosage of 50 Grays after surgery. Association with chemotherapy improves the response to radiotherapy [18].

The use of radiotherapy in patients already irradiated in the preoperative phase has long been discouraged due to the damaging effects that a second cycle of radiation may have on healthy tissue. In these patients, the maximum dose of radiation is 25 Grays. However, there are no studies comparing reradiated resected patients with resected patients who have not been reradiated [9].

15.6 Intraoperative Radiotherapy

Intraoperative radiotherapy (IORT) allows irradiation of the area of surgical interest, and may be used either in cases where the mass is not surgically removable or after the resection if there is some doubt regarding microscopic infiltration (R1).

The advantage of IORT is that it circumscribes the field to be irradiated, thus preserving the adjacent organs not infiltrated by the tumor.

The heterogeneity of the pattern of recurrence, the limited cases described in literature, and the absence of randomized prospective studies mean that we cannot at present express an opinion on the real benefits of IORT [19].

15.7 Surgical Therapy according to the Location

15.7.1 Axial Recurrences

Since the introduction of TME, the percentage of recurrences of the central compartment has dropped compared to the past.

In the event of strictly endoluminal recurrences without sphincter involvement, it is possible to perform an iterative anterior resection. Restoring bowel continuity must be discussed on the basis of the age of the patient, sphincter function and any reiterated radiotherapy. If an immediate anastomosis is deemed possible and safe, performing a J-pouch with loop-ileostomy is recommended. However, in a previously irradiated pelvis the functional results after a pouch are not excellent. If direct anastomosis is not indicated, a Hartmann operation can be performed.

Recurrences after abdominoperineal amputation must be treated with extensive exeresis (posterior or total exenteration) [20].

15.7.2 Anterior Recurrences

Anterior recurrences involve the adjacent pelvic organs like uterus and vagina in women, bladder, prostate and seminal vesicles in men.

In women, the presence of the uterus and the vagina preserve the bladder from neoplastic infiltration. In these cases an anterior exenteration with resection of the residual rectum, hysterectomy and partial or total colpectomy is possible. Vaginal resection may be repaired directly or with flaps.

In men, neoplastic invasion of the superior portion of the bladder may be treated with wedge resection and direct repair. More extensive infiltrations reaching the trigon of the bladder or involving the prostate are treated by total exenteration. In these cases the ureters are dissected where they cross the iliac vessels in order to preserve a sufficient length for urinary reconstruction. The dissection is carried out along the plane of the internal iliac vessels up to the elevator muscle plane.

After total exenteration, a urinary derivation must be prepared. The most frequently-used technique is the Bricker, an incontinent urinary diversion which consist in making an anastomosis between the last loop of the small bowel and the two ureters; subsequently an ileoileal anastomosis is required to restore digestive continuity. The irradiation of the distal small bowel loops often exposes the patient to the risk of anastomotic leakage. To reduce this risk, it is possible to use other intestinal segments, such as a portion of the duodenum or a section of the transverse colon.

It is currently possible to create continent urinary derivations by preparing a low-pressure reservoir using the right colon and the last ileal loops, whose functionality is guaranteed by the patient's self-catheterization. The aim of continent urinary derivations is to guarantee the patient an acceptable quality of life.

15.7.3 Posterior Recurrence

In 1981 Wanebo and Marcove [21] described for the first time abdominosacral amputation for posterior recurrences with infiltration of the pre-sacral fascia and of the sacrum, employing a technique already used for sarcomas and other mesenchymal tumors. In their first description, a laminectomy extending up to the S1-level was performed, with an attempt to preserve the S1-S2 nerve roots.

This procedure involves a high risk of nerve lesion with neurological consequences, as well as a high intraoperative mortality due to possible uncontrollable venous hemorrhage. Plastic surgery with buttock flap is necessary to restore the loss of substance. However, the healing process can be very difficult because of preoperative irradiation or the frequency of postoperative dehiscence and suppurations of the peritoneal cavity [22]. In the Wanebo case study, carried out on 53 patients, intraoperative mortality was 8%, the mean operative time was 20 hours with a mean blood loss exceeding 8,000 ml. The 5-year survival and disease-free survival rates were 31% and 23% respectively. For this reason, other authors have objected to this technique [12]. In 2004 Morya presented a case study of 57 patients subjected to exenteration with distal sacrectomy, limited at the bottom to the technically easier second sacral vertebra: the results showed a lower operative mortality rate (3.5%), a mean operative time of 682 minutes and almost half the blood loss (2,500 ml). Five-year survival rate was 46%, with fewer repercussions on a neurological level and an acceptable quality of life [23].

15.7.4 Lateral Recurrences

When the recurrence has a lateral extension, the possibility of performing an R0 resection decreases. The infiltration of the ureters and of the internal iliac arteries can be susceptible to resection with suitable reconstructions, while surgery for infiltration of the bony structures and of the sciatic nerve is not considered feasible.

15.8 Mortality and Morbidity

Postoperative mortality and morbidity are related to the type of operation performed. Mortality varies from 0 to 14%; higher postoperative mortality is reported for patients undergoing abdominosacral amputation [7].

The morbidity rates described in literature vary from 25 to 100%. The most frequent complications include pelvic abscesses (7-50%), intestinal obstructions (5-10%), enteric and urinary leakages (4-20%), perineal cavity suppurations (4-50%) and cardiac, renal and pulmonary complications. Abdominosacral amputations have a greater incidence of complications, with more than 50% occurring in the pelvic and peritoneal cavity. Transitory palsy of the sciatic nerve has also been reported, whatever the level of the sacral laminectomy [7].

Overall 5-year survival rates of patients undergoing R0, R1 and R2 resections ranges from 20 to 40%, with a mean survival rate from 24 to 32 months. The prognostic factor that most influences survival remains the radicality of the surgical resection, as demonstrated by the different case studies reporting a 5-yearsurvival rate ranging from 37 to 51% for R0 resections [7, 23, 24].

Patients with isolated anastomotic recurrence have a 5-year survival rate of 50% after R0 resection, while in some case reports the survival rate after R0 abdominosacral amputations varies between 30 and 40% [12], in spite of the high postoperative morbidity and mortality. The recurrence rate varies from 47 to 70% within 2 years [24].

15.9 Quality of Life

Miner et al. reported a reduction of pain and hemorrhages in the postoperative period in 78% of patients with symptomatic recurrence, with a mean recurrence of symptoms of 23 months, while 37% of patients with asymptomatic recurrence manifested pain in the postoperative period. In these cases, pain is usually due to sequelae of surgical trauma and to the outcome of the radiotherapy [25].

Multimodal treatment of recurrence produces consequences on patients' urinary and sexual functions. In particular, patients undergoing iterative anterior resection or abdominoperineal amputation may end up with urinary incontinence and impotence [26].

Patients with a dual by-pass seem to have an acceptable quality of life.

In abdominosacral amputations, section of S2-S3 nerve roots is the cause of vesical denervation and motor disturbances of the sciatic nerve, conditions susceptible to rehabilitation. The sexual function is preserved in the event of bilateral section of S3, while it is lost with monolateral section of S2. Monolateral section of the S1 roots causes walking problems due to deficit of the plantar flexion [12].

15.10 Conclusions

Local recurrence of rectal cancer leads to high morbidity for the patient. Radio- and chemotherapy can partially palliate the symptoms and extend the patient's life. Surgery remains the only option with a curative intent; however, it often results in significant morbidity and a decrease in the quality of life. It is therefore mandatory to select only patients eligible for curative surgery.

References

1. Abulafi AM, Williams NS (1995) Local recurrence of colorectal Cancer: the problem, mechanisms, management and adjuvant therapy. Br J Surg 81:7-19
2. Heriot AG, Kumar D (2000) Rectal Cancer recurrence: factors and mechanisms. Colorectal Dis 2:126-136
3. Van Lingen CP, Zeebregts CJ, Gerritsen JJ et al (2003) Local recurrence of rectal cancer after total mesorectal excision without preoperative radiotherapy. Int J Gastrointest Cancer 34:129-134

4. Sagar PM, Pemberton JH (1996) Surgical management of locally recurrent rectal cancer. Br J Surg. 83:296-304
5. Palmer G, Martling A, Cedemark B et al (2007) A population based study on the management and outcome in patients with locally recurrent rectal cancer. Ann Surg Oncol 14:447-454
6. Hahnloser D, Nelson H, Grunderson L et al (2003) Curative potential of multimodality therapy for locally recurrent rectal cancer. Ann Surg 237:502-508
7. Ghouti L, Portier G, Kirzin S, et al (2007) Traitment chirurgical des recidives locorégionales du cancer du rectum. Gastroenteral Clin Biol 31:55-67
8. Heriot AG, Tekkis PP, Darzi A et al (2006) Surgery for local recurrence of rectal cancer. Colorectal disease 8:733-747
9. Barkin J, Cohen M, Flaxman M (1988) Value of routine follow-up endoscopy for the detection of recurrent of colorectal cancer. Am J Gastroenterol 88:1355-60
10. Even Sapir E, Parag Y, Lerman H (2004) Detection of recurrence in patients with rectal cancer: PET/CT after abdominoperineal or anterior resection. Radiology 232:815-822
11. Sobin L, Wittekind C (1997) 5th Edition UICC International Union Against Cancer: TNM classification of malignant tumors. John Wiley and sons Inc, New York, p 67
12. Wanebo HJ, Antoniuk P, Koness RJ et al (1999) Pelvic resection of recurrent rectal cancer. Dis Colon Rectum 42:1438-1448
13. Yamada K, Ishizawa T, Niwa K et al (2001) Patterns of pelvic invasion are prognostic in the treatment of locally recurrent rectal cancer. Br J Surg 88:988-993
14. Guillem J, Ruo L (1998) Strategies in operative therapy for locally recurrent rectal cancer. Semin Colon Rectal Surg 9:259-268
15. Bropphy P, Hoffman J, Eisemberg B (1994) The role of palliative pelvic exenteration. Am J Surg 167:386-390
16. Khot U, Wenk Lang A, Murali K et al (2002) Systematic review of the clinical evidence on colo-rectal self expanding stents. Br J Surg 89:1098-1102
17. Farouk R, Nelson H, Gunderson LL (1997) Aggressive multimodality treatment for locally advanced irresectable rectal cancer. Br J Surg 84:741-749
18. Mohiuddin M, Hayne M, Regine WF et al (2000) Prognostic significance of postchemioradiation stage following preoperative chemotherapy and radiation for advanced recurrent rectal cancer. Int J Radiat Oncol Biol Phys 48:1075-1080
19. Wiig J, Poulsen J, Tveit K et al (2000) Intraoperative irradiation for primary advanced and recurrent rectal cancer: a need for randomised studies. Eur J Cancer 36:868-874
20. Houvenaeghel G (2002) Conservative surgery and restoration after pelvic exenteration. Bull Cancer 89:1061-1066
21. Wanebo HJ, Marcove RC (1981) Abdominal Sacral Resection of Locally Recurrent Rectal Cancer. Ann Surg 4: 458-471
22. Maetani S, Nishikawa T, Iijima Y et al (1992) Extensive en bloc resection of regionally recurrent carcinoma of the rectum. Cancer 69:2876-2883
23. Moriya Y, Akasu T, Fujita S et al (2004) Total pelvic exenteration with distal sacrectomy for fixed recurrent rectal cancer in the pelvis. Dis Colon Rectum 47:2047-2054
24. Boyle KM, Sagar PM, Chalmers AG et al (2005) Surgery for locally recurrent rectal cancer. Dis Colon Rectum 48:929-937
25. Miner TJ, Jacques DP, Paty PB et al (2003) Symptom control in patients with locally recurrent rectal cancer. Ann Surg 10:72-79
26. Mannaerts GH, Schijven MP, Hendrikx A et al (2001) Urologic and sexual morbidity following multimodality treatment for locally advanced primary and locally recurrent rectal cancer. Eur J Surg Oncol 27:265-272

Index

MIX
Papier aus verantwortungsvollen Quellen
Paper from responsible sources
FSC® C105338

If you have any concerns about our products,
you can contact us on
ProductSafety@springernature.com

In case Publisher is established outside the EU,
the EU authorized representative is:
Springer Nature Customer Service Center GmbH
Europaplatz 3, 69115 Heidelberg, Germany

Printed by Libri Plureos GmbH
in Hamburg, Germany